TANZANIAN DOCTOR

Tanzanian Doctor

by LEADER STIRLING

with an introduction by
JULIUS K. NYERERE
President of the United Republic of Tanzania

C. HURST & COMPANY · LONDON

First published in the United Kingdom by
C. Hurst & Co. (Publishers) Ltd.,
1-2 Henrietta Street, London WC2E 8PS

ISBN 0-903983-88-5

Printed in Great Britain by offset lithography by
Billing & Sons Ltd, Guildford, London and Worcester

To the Memory of my Mother,
who let Africa have me

Preface

This is not an autobiography, but the story of a young man who, more than forty years ago, was suddenly called to Africa from England and never went back. To serve God in Africa meant in fact to serve the people of Africa, and to serve the people of Africa it was necessary for him to become one of them, to sink his identity in a young nation, and to share their life, their troubles, their hopes and aspirations, and their struggle for health and freedom. These are the bones of the story. The following pages try to supply some of the flesh and blood.

The book has been written at odd times and in odd places, often on old bits of paper, and mostly without the help of a secretary. I am therefore deeply indebted to several very kind friends who did a lot of typing and put it into shape, especially Julia Carter, my brother-in-law Jerome Chisonga, my secretary Zaina Kombeson, and most of all my sister Audrey Holt-Wilson who, 6,000 miles away, did all the odd jobs and acted as my adviser and unofficial agent. I am also grateful to Richard and Alison Martin, to Frank Thorne and to my brother John for much valuable advice, and to Roger Lamburn for corrections on some facts of history, natural and otherwise. I thank the various photographers as named for the free use of their pictures. Those not attributed were taken by myself. Most of the people who come into the story appear with their real names, as they were all bits of history, and I hope they will forgive me.

Parts of Chapters II and X appeared many years ago in a collection of my letters borrowed and published by the Universities Mission to Central Africa. As I felt I could not improve on them for true description, and as they remained my property, I have included them with very slight alterations.

Lastly, my sincere thanks to Mwalimu Julius Nyerere, President of the United Republic of Tanzania, for so kindly providing the Introduction, and a word of thanks to my publisher, Christopher Hurst, for proving himself a skilled and sympathetic midwife.

Dar es Salaam, 1976 L. S.

Contents

Plates

Maps

Introduction

"There is no life of a man, faithfully recorded, but is a heroic poem of its sort, rhymed or unrhymed."

Thomas Carlyle

After 1967 the Tanzanian government made a great deal of noise about the need to take health services to the rural areas where the people lived. Until then government had, in practice, been allocating to urban medical care—and especially to Dar es Salaam—a large proportion of the meagre resources available. Thus, in 1969 for example, 22% of our health budget was being spent on one hospital in the capital city. Yet at that time only about 6% of the population lived in all the urban areas put together! Since then we have achieved some re-allocation of our public health expenditure, although once you have built a big consultant hospital—and we now have three—they have to be maintained and their heavy recurrent expenditures have to be met. We now estimate that 12.6% of the increased recurrent health budget is spent on Muhimbili hospital, and something like 67% is spent on rural medical services. Emphasis is given to providing preventive and curative medicine for the most common debilitating diseases like malaria and other fevers, and tuberculosis, as well as to mother and child care and mass immunization campaigns. Further, the urban hospitals have been better integrated into what is becoming a really national—although still very rudimentary—health service; the facilities of the major hospitals are therefore used for more complex treatment on reference from the rural centres, as well as serving people in the locality.

One of the many interesting things which is realised after reading this book is that, in adopting our new policy, we in Tanzania were not being nearly as new and revolutionary as our independent government imagined at that time. On the contrary we were, and are, continuing a tradition which seems to be as old as modern medical facilities in Tanzania. For example, the recent successful small-pox vaccination campaign, conducted with the help of WHO, was only doing on a more systematic basis and a larger scale what Dr. Stirling and his fellow-doctors and assistants were doing in the Masasi area some forty years ago—that is moving from village to village "vaccinating as we went".

The conditions of work were very much more difficult in the 1930s and '40s than they are now, despite all the restraints which still exist. Yet those difficulties were overcome with a spirit which should be an inspiration to all present day rural workers—in health and in other sectors of the economy. Thus, I am not sure how many of our present day workers would take for granted the need to walk for seven hours in order to reach a seriously injured patient, or the necessity to move from dispensary to dispensary by foot throughout the rainy season, and by bicycle at other times, when dispensaries were 20 to 30 miles from each other! But although such physical efforts are no longer demanded, the commitment to caring for people, and serving them at the cost of personal difficulty, is required as much in the 1970s as it was forty years ago.

Dr. Stirling's book has been directed mostly at a European audience, but it is a straightforward tale which is of great interest also to Tanzanians. I enjoyed reading it for many reasons. I have known Dr. Stirling for a long time, and my high opinion of his capacity, his attitudes and his dedication is indicated by his appointment as Minister for Health. But I know him better after reading this book; for without pretence or self-analysis, it is a description of the work he was doing, and the people and conditions he met throughout forty years of medical work in this country. And it is a book which reflects contentment in service. The complete absence of personal complaint, and the wry comments which cover what must often have been intense frustration, are an example to those of us who spend time complaining about all the things we cannot do because of shortage of resources or facilities.

But from reading *Tanzanian Doctor* I also caught a glimpse from a new angle of Tanzania's slow but steady progress. My home was in an area very different from those described by Dr. Stirling. But the lack of modern medical services which he describes existed in the Butiama I knew as a boy. We took their absence for granted. None of our people do so now.

And from the days when Dr Stirling walked 24 miles through the bush to his nearest subsidiary dispensary to the present day, when something like 90 per cent of our people live within 10 km. of a health facility, we have made advances in meeting the demands which have been aroused. It is the kind of advance which must encourage us to further efforts. For the facilities are neither common enough nor good enough.

We have to do still more training of workers and we have to expand medical facilities further. In doing this we have to maintain our priority of providing basic care near to the people rather than providing expensive treatment and facilities for the smaller number who suffer from less common diseases. This policy is rational and necessary. But for those who work in our hospitals it is not easy. The doctors of Tanzania, like those elesewhere in the world, are naturally reluctant to see people die in their hospitals when they know the treatment which could cure them but lack the facilities or the modern drugs to do it. Dr. Stirling's book illustrates, however, that this is not a new problem. And it shows also that progress can be made.

November 1976 JULIUS K. NYERERE

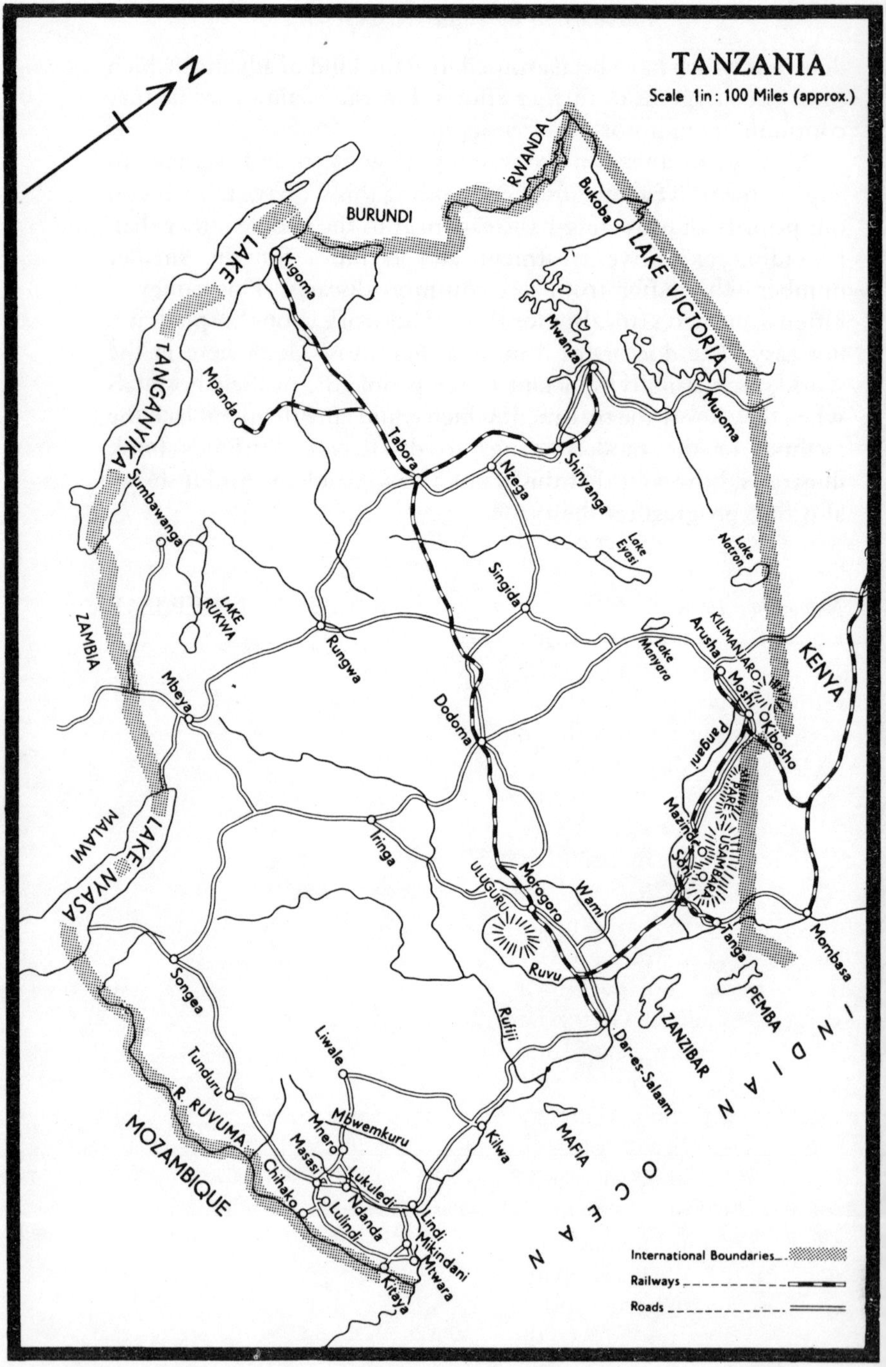
TANZANIA
Scale 1in : 100 Miles (approx.)
N
BURUNDI
RWANDA
Bukoba
LAKE VICTORIA
LAKE TANGANYIKA
Kigoma
Mwanza
Musoma
Mpanda
Tabora
Nzega
Shinyanga
Sumbawanga
Lake Eyasi
Lake Natron
LAKE RUKWA
Singida
ZAMBIA
Rungwa
KILIMANJARO
Arusha
Lake Manyara
KENYA
Moshi
Kibosho
Mbeya
Dodoma
Pangani
PARE
Mazinde
USAMBARA
MALAWI
LAKE NYASA
Iringa
ULUGURU
Morogoro
Wami
Tanga
Mombasa
Ruvu
PEMBA
Songea
Rufiji
ZANZIBAR
Dar-es-Salaam
INDIAN OCEAN
Liwale
Tunduru
R. RUVUMA
Mbwemkuru
Kilwa
MAFIA
MOZAMBIQUE
Mnero
Masasi
Lukuledi
Chihako
Lulindi
Ndanda
Lindi
Mikindani
Mtwara
Kitaya
International Boundaries
Railways
Roads

1

"Come over and help us"

London in the 1930s was a pleasant civilised place if you had a job, grim if you hadn't (the depression was on.) There was still room to walk down the street or cross the road. No speed limit, and park where you like. The trams were still clanging down the Whitechapel Road and along the Embankment and all over South London. Their drivers were my patients, among many others. Lunch in The London Hospital Club cost 1*s.* 4$\frac{1}{2}$*d.*, the fourpence-halfpenny being for a half-pint of Charrington's best bitter in a silver tankard, real beer out of a real barrel such as you seldom find now.

On the resident staff of the hospital we had excellent food and slept between linen sheets in comfortable rooms, but we had no salary. The appointment itself was considered a privilege, and in return for the privilege we were on call twenty-four hours a day, often working far into the night.

One warm May evening the night round was finished early, and about half-past ten I was brewing tea with my good friend and colleague, the late Dr. H. S. Atkinson. Henry said "Let's get out of this. I want to see bluebells". "Right", I said, "you've got the car, let's go." Henry's car was a nice two-seater sports model, and in no time we were zooming down the Whitechapel Road, through the empty City streets, over London Bridge and away. In half an hour we were on the North Downs, turning off at the top of Reigate Hill, down Gatton Lane, and up over Chaldon. We found them on the escarpment south of Woldingham, under the beech trees, seas of blue in the headlights. We loitered up and down the rough chalky lanes, Ganger's Hill, Little Hell, and the rest, just soaking in the beauty of the bluebells and the soft night air. Then we turned for London again, and by two o'clock we were back in bed and awaiting the next emergency. It was a great life.

I was born in England of an ancient Scots family, the eldest of four children. We grew up in the lovely Sussex Weald, with a very strong sense of home and family which we never lost. After primary education at a Catholic dame-school—St. Clare's, East Grinstead—I was sent to Bishops Stortford, one of the newer public schools, with a strongly radical and non-conformist tradition. The curriculum there showed a nice balance between the classics, modern science and languages, but we were perhaps unusual for those days in being taught philosophy, comparative religion, higher criticism and Einstein's theory of relativity. Many of our teachers were remarkable people, utterly dedicated to education in its deepest sense. I remember a lecture on leadership: leaders are born and not made, we were told, but we were sternly warned that every one of us must consider seriously whether we had not the gift of leadership, and if we had, it was our bounden duty to develop it with all the strength that God would give us. To allow the talent to lie buried was unforgivable.

Where the British Empire was concerned, the attitude at both schools was loyality, but with humility and no illusions, and a strong cultivation of self-criticism and the appreciation of human rights for all. Flag-wagging was strongly discouraged. One Empire Day the whole school was assembled in full expectation of being given a whole holiday. Instead of that we were given a severe lecture on the duty of self-effacing service, inner loyalty, and the utter impropriety of flag-waving. Then we were all sent back to our lessons.

To those two schools I owe more than I can say; they had a profound effect on my life which I only began to realise in later years.

My uncle was a doctor, my two cousins were doctors and so were my three great-uncles and even my great-grandfather, therefore from a very early age the practice of medicine seemed almost inevitable, and when I left school it was to read medicine at the University of London. Among my contemporaries were many students who professed rather loudly an intention of becoming medical missionaries, and most, though not all, fulfilled their intention. I was not one of them. As a boy I had been fairly intensively indoctrinated with missionary endeavour, especially by my grandmother, but while I admired the devotion and even heroism of the missionaries, I never felt the call myself. I always maintained that there was enough work to be done in England. Studying and working in London's East End, this was increasingly obvious as I got to know and love the people intimately, not only through obstetric work in their homes but through running a very tough troop of Boy Scouts there for six happy and exciting years.

After hospital I tried my hand at general practice, and found it equally fascinating. I too bought a car, an old coach-built Delage, what they called a "continental tourer". I paid £25 for it and had it painted racing green. It went like the wind, but my patients tolerated it.

Then I thought I would get back on the hospital ladder, and applied for several more senior appointments. I was short-listed for three and then the letter came out of the blue. It simply said "A doctor is urgently needed at Masasi. Can you go?" That was all. The address was the Universities' Mission to Central Africa. As I had been praying specially for guidance for the future only the day before, I could hardly ignore this obvious reply, so I wrote on a postcard "Yes, when?", and posted it quickly before I could have second thoughts.

I spent the rest of that day in the slightly intoxicated mood of one who had burned his boats, and next morning went to London to find out more about it. Masasi, I knew, was a pretty remote spot somewhere in Tanganyika, one of the centres of the U.M.C.A.'s activities. Beyond that I knew nothing. I found the Mission's London office and was kindly received. They outlined the situation briefly and again stressed its urgency. The only doctor at Masasi, a woman, was desperately overworked, with no prospect of relief. Two missionaries had died and several others had been invalided home; one without a leg—had been flown out of Masasi strapped onto the wing of a small plane. The health situation seemed bad, and the whole population depended on this one doctor. She must have help, quickly.

A ship was sailing in two weeks' time. Could I make it? The mood of elation was still strong and I would have liked to say "Yes", but natural caution was stronger. I saw several obvious difficulties, the most serious being that I knew next to nothing about tropical medicine. What little I knew had been gathered from the popular and stimulating, but all too short, course of lectures delivered annually by the great Manson-Bahr. The next ship after the first one was sailing a month later, which gave me six weeks to learn some more tropical medicine, and I agreed to sail on it. They gave me a paper to sign, which said that the first two years were a probationary period—after that anyone renewing was expected to do so with a life intention. The salary was £20 a year, all found. My father had always said "You needn't expect to make any money in medicine." In those days it was true. The Lord would provide. I signed.

Straightaway I began my preparations. I collected equipment and every day attended the London School of Hygiene and

Tropical Medicine, listening to lectures, peering down microscopes, making blood-films and picking up all I could. At the same time I pumped anyone I could find who knew anything about Masasi.

During these weeks I was also trying to learn Swahili, the lingua franca of East Africa. It seemed a reasonably easy language, with its neat constructions and absolute regularity of forms. I bought a grammar and began learning the numerals as I went home in the train. "*Moja, mbili, tatu nne . . .*"

I also began to find out more about the Universities' Mission to Central Africa. It had been founded in 1860, as the immediate response to an impassioned appeal by the great David Livingstone at the Senate House in Cambridge. Livingstone was, of course, a Presbyterian, but his co-religionists at that time were rather slow to rise to his appeal (they formed their own mission later), and he turned instead to the Anglican Church. The Universities' Mission was quickly formed, as a "mission to the Tribes around Lake Nyassa". from the beginning the mission was organised on a high-church basis, in the tradition of the Tractarians, and was placed under the autocratic leadership of a bishop specially consecrated for the task. As the years passed the high-church tradition gradually developed into a more and more extreme "Anglo-Catholic" position, until the Mission was propagating a religion which bore little outward resemblance to that of the Church of England as usually understood.

From early days the members of the Mission, clerical and lay alike, were bound by a written promise of celibacy and obedience to the Bishop. Poverty was not included in the promise, but was effectively achieved by providing only the simplest board and lodging, on a communal basis, and paying no salary. Pocket money was issued at £18 a year, "if necessary", and a small outfit allowance every three years. It was often said that only a person with private means could survive in the mission, but a number of us without managed all the same.

The Mission nearly died at birth, the first bishop and several of his small company dying of malaria and dysentry within a few months of landing on the Zambezi. After some anxious years of retreat and reorganization, however, it had become well established in Zanzibar, on the shores of Lake Nyasa, and in the north and south of Tanganyika. Much later a further advance was made into what is now Zambia.

The Mission attracted some very able and utterly devoted men and women, mostly university graduates, many of whom died on the job after few or many years' service. Several served the African Church for more than fifty years. The Community of the Sacred Passion, an order of professed nuns under perpetual vows, founded by the saintly Bishop Weston of Zanzibar, worked in and with the Mission with amazing devotion and are still active, some at great age.

The chief activity of the Mission, apart from direct evangelism, was always education, in which they were among the most effective pioneers in many regions. The literacy rate in remote Masasi District, the highest in all Tanzania, is primarily the fruit of their labours. Medical work was also promoted from the earliest years, and eventually became a wide-spread and well organised service in the spreading of the Gospel, although the medical workers available were never equal to the ever-growing demands. This was where I came in.

Because of its theological position, the Mission had always been rather vulnerable to the claims of the Catholic Church, and from early days there was a sporadic trickle of defections. After 1945 the trickle became a stream and in the next ten years or so eighteen members of the Mission who had resigned made their submission to Rome. This inevitably produced a reaction; a slight but definite retreat from the extreme Anglo-Catholic position. There was a trimming of sails in a more recognisably Anglican direction, which was further encouraged by the very necessary movement for closer union with the other Anglican missions, notably the Church Missionary Society whose theological position was poles apart from U.M.C.A.

Eventually the Universities' Mission was absorbed into the Society for the Propagation of the Gospel, which marked the union by prefixing the word "United". This was probably necessary for reasons of manpower and finance, but many regretted the passing of what was in many ways a unique institution which made a notable contribution to both the evangelisation and development of Tanzania.

Meanwhile my time was short, and after a round of farewell visits I tore up my roots and sailed from Tilbury on 21 March 1935, a beautiful spring day. A friend had remarked casually, "So you're sailing on St. Benedict's day. He's a good one to look after you." Casual or not, those were prophetic words. The ship sailed smoothly down the Thames in the evening calm. I looked back into the sunset where my mother, my sister and my little niece were becoming ever smaller on the landing-stage. England was disappearing into the darkness and into the time of days-gone-by, officially for two years but in fact for ever.

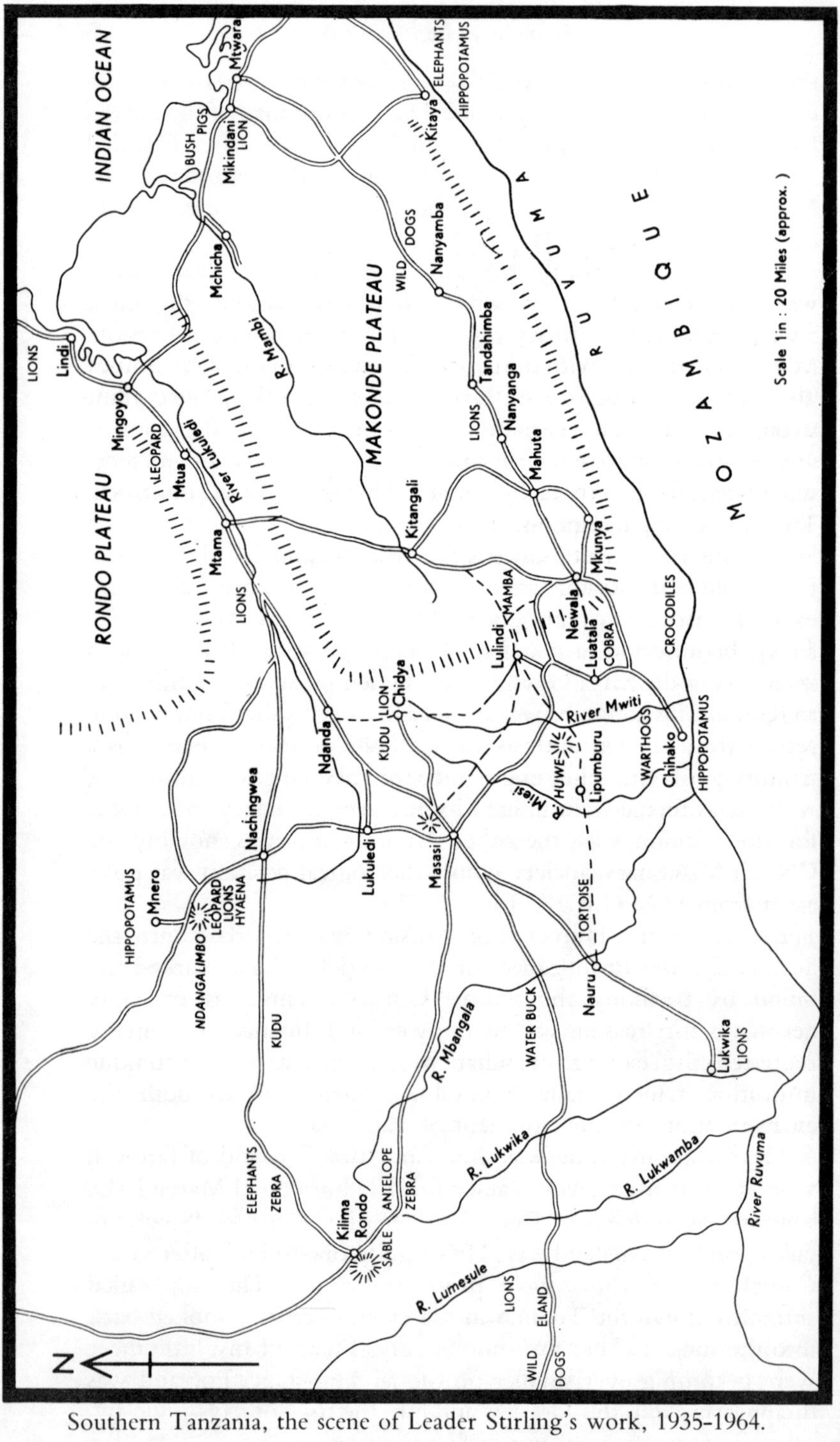

Southern Tanzania, the scene of Leader Stirling's work, 1935-1964.

2
The Road to Masasi

Four weeks later I landed in Zanzibar. The heat and sunlight, contrasting fiercely with the cool dark interiors of old Arab houses, the narrow twisting streets, the cheerful people, the all-pervading aroma, at once rich, fascinating and repulsive—the riotous green foliage, the flowers and fruits, the loud nocturnal chorus of frogs and insects, the rain that falls with a solid roar and stops abruptly to leave a steaming dampness, and always the brilliant, clear sea, with white sands and white-sailed boats; that is Zanzibar.

I stayed at the headquarters of the Mission, and was made very welcome. Someone said, "This is Francis, he will look after you." Francis smiled and held out his black hand and suddenly I had a qualm of misgiving. I had never had any contact with Africans before, and I thought "What if I find myself quite incompatible with them?" It was unthinkable yet there it was, and there was Francis, smiling and holding out his hand; I could not hesitate, and with an irrational feeling that the black would come off, I took it. In that grip misgiving vanished and a great door opened.

I stayed in Zanzibar over Easter, and waited for the steamer that would carry me down the Tanganyika coast. The *Dumra* was small and slow, but clean and comfortable. It carried few passengers and little cargo, so we rolled heavily. After Dar es Salaam I was the only second-class passenger. We called at small unknown ports— a few palm-thatched huts between the bush and the sea— where we lay well off the coral reefs and sandy beaches. Cargo was ferried to and fro in primitive sailing boats or an ancient lighter. No one was in a hurry.

On the third day we entered Lindi Bay and anchored in the mouth of a wide creek. From the sea Lindi had an attractive appearance. Across the blue water of the bay the long curve of white sand, and beyond it palm trees and a sprinkling of neat white buildings some with red roofs, gave an ideal picture of tropical Africa. We went ashore in a motor-boat, and the illusion rapidly disappeared. After half an hour I had seen Lindi, and it was a dump.

I was met by the Mission's local agent, a Goanese general dealer.

He was lean and yellow, with an old topee, and seemed permanently tired. He never spoke unless spoken to, and seemed to take life sadly, perhaps the result of living in Lindi. His shop seemed to stock little and sell less. However, he sold me a pair of shoe-laces, which immediately broke, and told me I could start by motor-boat next morning for Masasi. Meanwhile he produced some food, and I spent the night in an old shed by the shore that was euphemistically described as the Mission rest-house. However, I was well looked after by an elderly African servant who had been sent from Masasi to escort me. I had learnt from a letter that his name was Daudi, so calling up all the Swahili I knew, I asked him "*Wewe* Daudi?". He smiled and replied "*Ndiyo, Bwana*". ("You Daudi?" "Yes Sir.") From this simple exchange sprang a legend that I had landed at Lindi speaking fluent Swahili.

Daudi had retired from Mission service, but had been called out to receive the newcomer. He was quiet, cheerful and imperturbable, and looked after me well. He wore the white *kanzu,* an Arab garment rather like a Victorian nighshirt, which was then still something of a status symbol but also, strangely, the regular dress of a domestic servant (like the English waiter's black bow-tie). It is still popular with Muslims, much as the frock-coat in England lingered on among the Non-conformists, but otherwise it has almost disappeared.

At seven next morning we embarked in a motor-boat and started up the river on the tide. I had been told in London that the boat would take me the first twenty miles and that I should then have to walk the remaining seventy-five. However, to my relief, I heard that a lorry had been chartered and hoped to get through. It would be the first of the season. The rains had just ended, and much of the country was still water-logged, but it was thought the "main road" would now be passable.

As the wind was against the tide, the river was choppy and plenty of spray came into the boat. After about an hour and a half it suddenly dwindled to a muddy winding creek, and we stopped at a small wharf. Presently a lorry appeared, and my luggage was loaded on to it. We climbed a short hill into a village of Mingoyo and stopped there while the driver, an Indian, prepared for the journey. He loaded on a large jack, a shovel, a spare radiator and a breakdown crew of four or five Africans, besides a few casual passengers. I had the wooden seat beside him, and after a long delay we set off. We crashed and bumped along. The road varied considerably—from fair to unspeakably bad—but nowhere was it metalled. I was comfortable enough in front, but was sorry for the crew behind me, on the floor among the boxes. About midday we stopped at Mtama, an untidy village with some dilapidated Indian shops, and I ate a lunch of sandwiches. The driver ordered a large meal of curried chicken and rice, in which he pressed me to join him, so I had a second lunch. Meanwhile the crew were busy changing the radiator. The original one had been leaking so fast that it was permanently boiling and had to be filled every mile or so. The new one was a lot better: it lasted at least three miles, or perhaps even five, without a refill.

In the afternoon we travelled steadily inland. We had left the sisal plantations and were now in natural bush country, green and pleasant—but not exciting. On a steep hill we stuck in the loose earth, but by putting roadside grass in the tracks and all pushing, we were soon moving on. At four o'clock we stopped at Ndanda, the headquarters of the Catholic Mission in those parts, a Benedicitine foundation with an Abbot-Bishop and a small community of Fathers, Brothers and Sisters. I was hospitably received and given tea by the late Sister Thekla Stinnesback, who was the only doctor between Masasi and the coast, and already a legend in her own lifetime. She showed me over her busy hospital and was both kind and encouraging, and informative. She also introduced me to some of the fathers. I felt I had friends already. St. Benedict was at work!

At last the driver, afraid that we would be benighted, began to agitate for a move. So reluctantly and with many kind messages for the Mission at Masasi, we set off again. After Ndanda the road became worse. Bridges, previously insecure, now became non-existent, and we traversed frequent fords. Twice we stuck utterly, with the back wheels axle-deep in mud. Then the crew got busy with the jack and shovel and dug us out. At a narrow place we passed another lorry, the only traffic all day. There was just room for two lorries, but not for the hurricane lamps that our driver had tied to the side for safety. They were simply stripped off and pulverised with a rending crash, but we did not stop. The driver simply shouted "Both?" and when someone behind shouted back "Yes, both", he shrugged his shoulders and drove on. We had still some miles to go when darkness fell, and the driver pressed on at increased speed. The pot-holes in the road were often invisible in the dark and it seemed a wonder that we had any springs or axles left. Then we began to run through long grass, higher than the radiator, and could see nothing at all. Every minute I expected that we would plunge headlong into a hidden chasm, but at last the dim outline of the mountain began to break the skyline and presently we reached a single hut which was the beginning of Masasi. A few yards further on one of our right wheels was suddenly snared by a treacherous patch of bog and sank deeply. In a moment the lorry had slewed round and turned over in the ditch. The driver threw up his hands and screamed, but we remained firmly embedded, undamaged but at an angle of 45 degrees. I jumped out and Daudi touched my arm and using all his English said "Let us go". We walked briskly up the hill in the dark for half a mile, and surprised the mission staff at dinner. Apparently they had not really believed that the lorry would get through. But I was soon made at home by the Vicar-General (later Bishop F. O. Thorne of Malawi), and after a week he could say "I feel you've always been here."

3

I walk to Lulindi

I found Masasi a place to dream of. A great mountain rises straight up behind the Mission, steep green wooded slopes crowned with a sheer rocky precipice. Two buttresses of the mountain stand out on either side, curving round almost in a semi-circle like protecting wings. Below, a vast sea of rolling bush—green, gold, blue of a hundred shades in the ever-changing light, studded with rocky islands—is bounded by distant lines of great blue hills.

In the centre of the Mission was the cathedral, a long building in rough-hewn stone, impressive in its simplicity. Around it were grouped the houses of the missionaries, simple mud huts in ordinary African style, thatched with grass. This was the pattern throughout the diocese, and away from Masasi itself even the churches were built in the same style of mud and thatch. The Bishop was very keen on this, as he felt that it lessened the gulf between the African people and the missionaries and made them feel more at home in church. This was true enough, but with rapidly advancing education it began to look to some Africans as though the Mission were trying to retard their material progress. Anyway, for the next fourteen years I was to live in a mud hut, and I found it cool and comfortable.

The first person I met at Masasi was Dr. Frances Taylor, an indomitable woman, in equal parts steel and devotion, who was in charge of the medical work. She outlined its scope. Here at Masasi she had a general hospital, staffed with two English trained nurses and a number of locally trained dressers. In the surrounding country she had the care of six similar but smaller hospitals, half a dozen dispensaries scattered through the remoter parts of the bush, and two leprosy settlements. Besides this she was responsible for the health of the mission staff and the children in the various boarding schools. From one end of her district to the other was over 200 miles, and the roads were impassible to wheeled traffic for five months every year. Then she would walk or swim when necessary, endless journeys of 20-30 miles a day, constantly being called from one hospital to another to the latest emergency, rarely able to settle down to constructive work in peace, and rarely having more than three hours' sleep a night. In her district there was no other doctor. Private practitioners did not exist, and the nearest government medical officer was anchored at Lindi 95 miles away. For a time she had a colleague, but the colleague did not last long and she was alone again. For nine years she had carried on like this, and the situation was becoming impossible. Several of the missionaries were seriously ill, two had recently died, one had acquired leprosy and half a dozen had been invalided home. She herself had often been sick. Hence the urgent appeal I had received.

Masasi hospital itself was in a primative state. The outpatient building was a thatched hut of *pisé-de-terre,* in the middle of which sat the doctor or a nurse, surrounded by a solid throng of pushing humanity. But each patient's particulars were carefully entered, his fee collected, usually in grain or cassava, eggs, vegetables, a hen, a bottle of honey or a roll of tobacco, and a diagnosis made. The senior nurse, Florence Smith, kept up a stream of instructions in an extraordinary mixture of three languages, miraculously bringing order out of imminent chaos and keeping everyone laughing. As the patients were dealt with they were separated into different corners of the room according to the different treatments they needed. In each corner a dresser stood ready, treating them one by one and telling them when to come again. Dressings and injections were given in a seperate hut, a flimsy structure of bamboo and grass, and a similar building served as a laboratory. As one worked at the microscope by the open window, snakes and lizards moved around outside, or even inside, and brightly coloured birds flew in and out.

The inpatients were housed in small mud huts holding two or three beds apiece. These huts straggled all down the hillside, like a rather untidy village. The patients' relatives lived with them in the huts, sleeping on the floor and cooking for them outside in an open shelter. They would rather have cooked in the huts, but that was forbidden. However the cooking pots and stores of food, live hens, spears and bows and arrows were stored under the patients' beds.

There was an operating theatre too. It was another open-work bamboo building with a grass roof, and every gust of wind filled it with dust and dead leaves. A hen had also found its way in between the bamboos and was nesting quietly in a corner. There was no running water in the hospital, and no lighting except for oil lamps. There was no heat sterilization except for operations, when a pair of large primus stoves were lit. Otherwise everything was done, or not done, by lysol and faith. If hot water was needed, someone went to beg a little from the kitchen. There was of course no X-ray.

Meeting an efficient English nurse whom I had known at the London Hospital, I asked her how she could reconcile herself to such appalling conditions. "Oh", she said "this is Africa and so one must accept lower standards." I was so shocked by this reply that I determined I would never accept any lowering of standards. Of facilities, yes—one had to make the best of what one could get—but standards, no! And it is surprising what can be achieved with the most primitive facilities if there is insistence on keeping standards. Edith Shelley, of whom I shall say much more later, was a nurse who was often criticised by her smarter colleagues for her apparent carelessness and rough and ready simplicity, yet in fact by her practical ability and resourcefulness she achieved with the simplest equipment higher standards of nursing care and asepsis than they did.

In these conditions more than 1,000 new admissions and 5,000 new outpatients were dealt with in a year. A normal day's work entailed some 300 treatments. Conditions in the other hospitals were similar, except that in the absence of the doctor the whole responsibility fell on the senior (or sometimes only) nurse, even to the extent of her performing emergency operations such as amputations after wild-beast injuries. Two nurses once succeeded in cutting off a leg, but could not find the femoral artery to tie it—however, the patient recovered. In general the results were very good.

Once when I was visiting the hospital of another mission, the doctor showed me a rather primitive outpatient building, contrasting badly with the pleasant rooms provided for sick missionaries. "Good enough for the natives", she remarked quite casually. "Good enough" implies that there is a reasonable limit to charity, but St. Paul didn't think so. I began to realise that I had to contend not only with the devil and disease, but with the shocking prejudices of some of my senior colleagues. Another said flatly "All Africans have bugs, even the cleanest of them", a preposterous statement that I found totally false. (There are plenty of bugs in Africa, if you know where to look for them, but so there were in England when I worked there.)

In the cathedral a cross in the floor marked the grave of Canon William Porter. He had been a pioneer missionary in the nineteenth and early twentieth centuries, and had become a legend. He was very tough. Once in his earlier days he had gone alone and unarmed to bargain with the fierce Angoni raiders for the return of the people they had carried off from the Christian village of Masasi. He got them all back unhurt. He was said to have found the station at Masasi uncongenial, so he spent most of his time out in the bush, walking all day and visiting people in their villages. He went by himself on foot and took no food, but in the pocket of his cassock, which he always wore, he carried a small tin of tea, a tin mug and a spirit lamp. When he became too weary he would stop in the forest, light his little spirit lamp, and brew himself black tea. He was greatly loved, and on one occasion as he entered a village a small child ran crying to its mother, "There's a European!" "Stupid" said mother, "that's no European, that's a-Porter!"

There is a story that on another occasion he was travelling with the Archdeacon of Masasi and they slept in a village school with an open doorway. In the middle of the night Porter was awakened by the Archdeacon calling in a hoarse whisper, "Porter, Porter!" "Eh?" "There's a leopard under your bed!" "What's that?" The Archdeacon (rather louder). "There's a *Leopard under your bed!*" Porter (slowly turning over and peering under the bed): "Look here, you can't come in here. *Get out!*" The leopard got out, and Porter turned over and went to sleep again.

To escape from Masasi, Porter moved out to Lumesule, some seventy miles to the west and laboured there alone until his death in 1908. He was later buried in the cathedral at Masasi with the honours due to a saint.

After a week or two at Masasi, Dr. Taylor began showing me the district. One of the first places we visited was Lulindi, as this was to be my headquarters. The Lulindi road was still impassible, so we set out on foot at 3 a.m. and walked twenty-four miles through the bush. I enjoyed the novelty of it then—fording streams in the dark, the endless vista of the forest in the cool dawn, the orange sun coming up over the hills. But after doing it some fifteen times I was thankful when at last the road became motorable at all seasons.

The country we passed through was all forest and bush with scattered hamlets, one every few miles. Each hamlet of two or three huts was surrounded by its fields of millet and beans, and there were usually some meagre hens. The people are entirely agricultural, and make their fields by clearing and . . . burning the forest. The soil is often poor, and the ash from the burning was then the only enrichment if ever received. After two years it was exhausted, and the family had to make new fields. If they had a death, or even much sickness, or bad harvests, they would move altogether and build a new village at a distance, to get away from the influence of local spirits or of their neighbours, who might be thought to have caused the trouble by charms, spells, and poisons. In this way the shape of the countryside was constantly changing. Familiar villages quietly disappeared and were eaten up by the ever-hungry bush, while new clearings and new huts appeared elsewhere. (The Ujamaa villages have changed all that.)

There was no European settlement. Apart from the missionaries the only Europeans in the country were the Government officials, and at that time there was only one of these at each of the smaller Government stations, which were about a hundred miles apart. Masasi was one such, the *boma*★ being about three miles from the Mission. Masasi had a telegraph, but it was the end of the wire. The next three *bomas* had no means of communication with each other and the outside world except runners (why so-called I cannot imagine as I have never seen one attempting to run).

The last mile into Lulindi was through thick sand and slightly uphill, and the sweat began to trickle down my back. We arrived at 10.30.

★*Boma* = (originally) a stockade, but now simply a Government post.

4

Up on the Plateau

I liked Lulindi. It was a comparatively new station and the work was growing streadily. There was a cheerful, friendly atmosphere and an absence of that mildew of the past that tends to cling to older mission stations. It was also free of the self-conscious busyness that afflicts headquarters stations. The climate was pleasant with bright dry days and cool nights even in hot weather, as the hotter the day the more cold air poured down at night from the high Makonde Plateau three miles away. There were big shady trees and bright flowers. Fruit was plentiful and there was a vegetable garden. The chief had a small herd of cows—quite a rarity in those days—which gave some milk. For meat we had fowls,. a duck on Sundays, and sometimes a goat or sheep for special occasions. Other supplies had to come from Lindi, and from time to time a gang of porters set off for the 200-mile walk, bringing it all back on their heads. They used to earn four or five shillings each, a sum which in those days would feed a man for six weeks, or buy him a shirt and loincloth, or pay his tax for a year.

I was accommodated in a small hut to which I at once took a great liking. It had one room, a large verandah, and a pleasant outlook towards the hills. I later added a second room and had it re-thatched. It was very simple: there was no ceiling and the windows had no glass. They were just holes punched out of the mud and barred over with a few bamboos. The floor was beaten earth, with a few palm-leaf mats. For light I had an ordinary paraffin hurricane lantern, such as were then used in England for marking road obstructions at night. By bringing it right close to my book or paper, and turning the wick up full, I manged to work long hours after the hospital had settled for the night. Water was brought in a four-gallon petrol tin from the stream half a mile away, and I had an old Victorian hip-bath which I could use either on the bedroom floor or in the backyard, which was fenced round with grass, with a gap leading to a pit-latrine. My bed was of the ordinary African

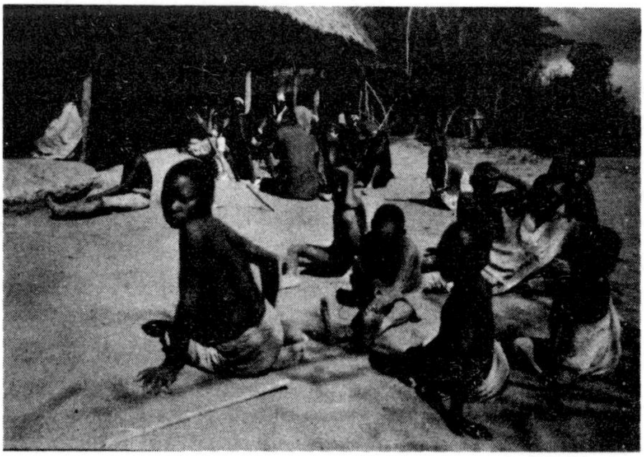

Above, Newala dispensary with outpatients waiting to be seen.

Below, the old ambulance on the road to Lulindi.

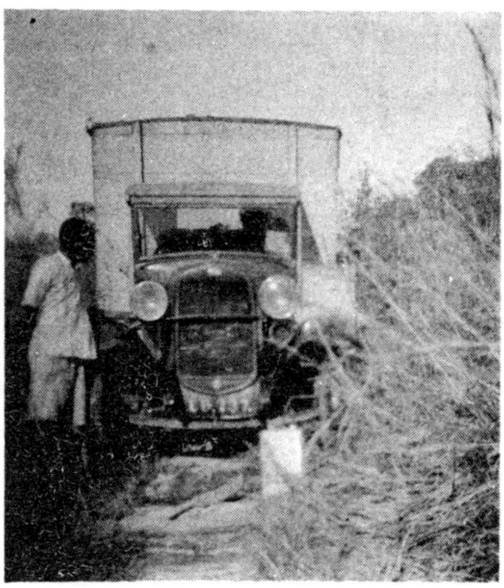

type, a light wooden frame strung with a palm-leaf rope covered by a palm-leaf mat, on which I slept soundly without a mattress for nearly thirty years.

This hut was my home for fourteen happy years. At this time, however, I could not yet settle at Lulindi, as I had the rest of the district to see, and after about a week we moved on to Newala. Dr. Taylor meanwhile had walked back to Masasi and had managed to get the Mission ambulance through to Lulindi, as the roads were now drying out and were being repaired. The ambulance was locally built on the chassis of a $1\frac{1}{2}$-ton "Model B" Ford with a second-hand engine. It was very roomy, but the body swayed and creaked at every bump, and except when it was very well loaded it seemed to have no springs at all. When transporting a patient it was necessary to ballast it with sacks of salt or sand. However, it was easier than walking, and after battling with some heavy sand and repeatedly refilling the boiling radiator we eventually climbed the 1000 feet on to the Makonde Plateau. Once there we had dry roads in good condition and were able to visit dispensaries in the ambulance.

The plateau country was something new. Nearly all the primeval forest had disappeared and been replaced by an endless expanse of secondary bush. This was so dense that only a wild pig could penetrate it, and growing to a height of ten feet or more it effectively shut out all view of the surrounding country from the slot-like paths and roads. The paths tended to become tunnels. One could drive for miles through this bush without sight of a house, thus having the quite false impression that the country was uninhabited. Actually the bush was honeycombed with paths leading to hamlets in small clearings, and was one of the most densely populated areas in Tanganyika.

The greater altitude made the climate cooler, and at night the clouds came down, drenching the vegetation and making the mornings bitterly cold. There was an almost total absence of water on the plateau as the soil was too porous to allow it to collect anywhere. Consequently every drop of water had to be carried up from the valley 1,000 feet below, and a familiar and striking sight was a procession of rapidly moving scantily clad figures in the bitter cold of early dawn, carrying gourds of every size and shape down to the wells, and toiling back fully laden many hours later. Those who lived only an hour from the escarpment regarded the water as "near". Some came as far as ten miles to the escarpment, and still had the 1,000 foot descent to the water—and then the journey back. Such people would set out for the wells at three in the morning in order to be home by mid-day. A grown woman would carry three full gourds of water—one hung on each end of a pole over her shoulder, and the third one balanced on her head. As a large gourd may hold up to five gallons, a strong woman could be carrying a weight of up to 150 lbs., first up a 1,000-foot climb so steep that handholds are needed in some places, and then for ten miles of dusty path to the village. Each person carries what he or she can, the children following their elders with gourds of diminishing size, until at the end comes a quite small child proudly balancing a precious pint on its head.

To live under such conditions day after day and year after year would appear intolerable, but the Makonde people are tough and obstinate, and the need for water did no more than determine their pattern of life. The traditional scheme was for the women of the village to go to the well one day and the men the next. On the third day nobody went; the family simply went dry. Water was consequently for cooking only, except when beer was to be made. Little was drunk and none was used for washing. All bathing and the washing of clothes was done while at the wells, which thereby became the great social meeting places where news was exchanged and goods bartered while the clothes were drying and the water-pots filled. After the long walk and the waiting, these crowds of people of course performed their natural functions in the immediate surroundings of the wells, thereby contaminating the wet soil with hookworm larvae, and infecting each other with great rapidity. This accounted for the paradox that hookworm infestation, which requires wet earth for its transmission, is commoner and more serious in degree among the people of the waterless plateau than among many of the valley dwellers. On the other hand bilharzia, so prevalent in the valleys, is unknown on the plateau, as infection normally requires fairly prolonged immersion in infested water and the wells of the Wamakonde are far too precious for paddling. (Bilharzia does occur on the plateau but only in those rare places where pools of water occur in pockets of clay.)

The Wamakonde explain their living at such an inconvenient distance from water by a tribal taboo, but it is more likely that this story was conveniently invented after they had taken refuge on the plateau from warlike tribes, and so had perforce become cut off from water. In any case the alleged taboo is conveniently forgotton in these days when at last the water problem is being reluctantly tackled on a big scale, and the Government has brought piped water from the valley to all parts of the thirsty plateau.

In spite of the lack of water, the plateau is remarkably fertile, being watered by the clouds and drenching dews. The Wamakonde get three seasons from a field, against only two in the valley. They grow maize, cassava and hill-rice, all of which were formerly sold for cash, the people living on wild roots only. How they spent their money was a mystery, as they wore few clothes and had none of the trappings of 'civilisation'. Probably it was buried. Things have changed now. The young men returning from the Second World War demanded something better than roots and a loincloth, and the Wamakonde are using their money, as well as eating some of their own crops.

The medical situation at Newala was somewhat different from that at Masasi and Lulindi. In the first place the old missionary in charge of the station (the late Canon F. W. Stokes) would not allow any proper hospital to be built, as he feared it might be seen as 'bribery' for the Faith. He permitted a dispensary, and to this the sick came in their hundreds. Those who were too ill to go home after treatment had to be accommodated down the road in a hutted camp maintained by local government. Many were too ill to walk, so the Sister in charge of the dispensary and her two dressers had to make frequent visits out to the camp to treat them as they lay. On my first day there a boy was carried in with a broken thigh-bone. There was no extension apparatus, so I had to improvise, making a Thomas' splint of bamboo and baling iron, and for pulleys using the empty reels of adhesive plaster. This contraption we slung up to wooden posts driven into the earth floor of the hut, and there the boy was nursed until his bone was sound. This was only the beginning of improvisation, and I soon found how much conventional surgical equipment can be dispensed with when necessity so dictates.

This hutted camp was a well-intentioned idea, but the local government had no medical staff to supervise it properly and our Sister had no authority there. There was just an old man with a wooden leg who used to sweep it out and keep some sort of order. This did not prevent lodgers from a distance from bringing in ticks (*ornithodorus moubata*) heavily infected with *spirillum Duttoni,* the causative organism of East African relapsing fever. These ticks multiplied unchecked and unknown to the dispensary staff, until the father of a sick child was found unconscious with a high fever. The Sister took blood films and examined them, but did not know what to make of them. She was, after all, only a nurse, and tick fever was rare at Newala. She sent urgently for me, twenty miles away. I came at once, but even so the poor man was already dead. I looked down the waiting microscope: ten spirilla in the first field!

Running a camp or hostel for patients' relatives is a grave responsibility. On another occasion at Lulindi the father of a sick child thought he would take the chance to have some medicine. He was examined, found to have hookworm, and duly dosed. Not content, he came again the next morning. It was Sunday, with minimum staff, and an untrained assistant was giving out some routine mixtures with which he could do no harm. Finding that the old man had had oil of chenopodium the previous day, he fetched the bottle, without any authority, and measured him a liberal half-ounce, i.e. fifteen times the normal dose. The poor old man was soon unconscious on the floor, and I spent the whole of Sunday morning washing out his stomach and trying to revive him, but it was too much and he died.

Another notable difference at Newala was the much greater prevalence of yaws. This is a horrible disease beginning with a foul ulcer in some part, usually the leg, and continuing with tumid sores all over the body. Later, deep ulcers break out in different parts, bones ache, swell and rot away; sometimes a large part of the nose and mouth may be destroyed. After many years the disease eventually dies out, leaving the victim more or less scarred and crippled. With injections of arsenic, bismuth or penicillin the disease can be cut short at any stage and permanently cured. (The dramatic effect on yaws of bismuth injections, the first cheap and simple remedy, probably started the East African vogue for injections as the cure for everything.) Nevertheless at that time it was still all too common in many places, partly because hospitals were so inaccessible but more because of the lack of persistence on the part of the patients. After one or two injections they would see such a dramatic improvement that they were quite satisfied, and no words would persuade them to continue with treatment until they were fully cured. So the disease smouldered on and infection continued to spread. It has now, however, disappeared with the use of long-acting penicillin.

At that time the Makonde plateau was still full of yaws, and day after day the dispensaries were crowded with sufferers at every stage of the disease, some pictures of sheer horror such as I have not seen elsewhere, confluent sores literally from head to foot, sometimes a gaping hole where the face had been, or a leg hanging by the skin only.

There was another dispensary a dozen miles away at Mahuta where the situation was even worse, and to deal more thoroughly with the problem I opened three more dispensaries on the plateau in the next few years. Three years later the old missionary had retired to a smaller station, and I was able to begin building a hospital at Newala.

The Wamakonde were less frightened of surgery than the other tribes, and on the first visit I was already able to operate on a child with chronic osteomyelitis of the leg, removing a loose piece of dead bone the size of a banana. I had previously only seen such things in museums.

After barely a week came the inevitable urgent recall to Masasi. This time it was an epidemic of small pox which had just come to light. It had apparently been concealed in the bush for weeks, and there was no idea yet how extensive it might be. Regretfully leaving the cool plateau we returned in haste to Masasi.

5
Smallpox in the Bush

For the next three months smallpox dominated everything. Our ordinary work was dislocated and every day was a long trail through the bush, looking for cases, following up rumours, arranging the isolation of patients and treating them in their distant isolations. We found and treated over 200 cases, and in the first two weeks vaccinated more than 10,000 contacts and neighbours. For the vaccinating we had the help of a team of our dressers, but diagnosis of cases and later their certification of discharge needed the visit of a doctor, as well as interim visits to check progress. So day after day Dr. Taylor and I were out, often from morning till evening, each in a different direction, walking from village to village and from the villages to isolation camps far into the bush. We vaccinated as we went and gave what simple treatment we could to the patients to relieve their symptoms and prevent complications. There is of course no specific treatment to cut short an attack of smallpox. To our great relief, however, the epidemic proved a mild one, and only two patients died (one of these deaths was due to an isolation hut catching fire).

Although this endless foot-slogging, day after day through the mid-day heat, was rather tiring, it gave me a close and concentrated introduction to the country, the villages, the people and the flora and fauna that I might otherwise not have obtained in years. I learnt to follow the forest paths and to distinguish the path to the well, the path to the fields and the path to the village. There were new trees, new flowers, strange birds, small animals and curious reptiles and insects everywhere. One day I suddenly saw an animal almost the size of a horse standing motionless a few yards ahead. It was a fine bull kudu with magnificent spiral horns and mane. I stood still in wonder and then some yards behind I saw two pairs of huge ears twitching, where his wives were lurking among the bushes.

Most valuable of all was the practice in talking Swahili. Meeting only Africans all day and having to ask my way, enquire about patients and give instructions was worth more than months of work with a book.

When following reports of new cases, I usually had a schoolboy or young man from the nearest village as a guide. On one such search we had walked several fruitless miles in the midday heat, and stopped to rest. I unslung my water bottle, and my young guide begged a drink. I handed it to him and he had a good pull. It seemed the obvious and natural thing to do, but I realised some of my superiors would have been shocked. "Sharing your water-bottle with an African!" However they weren't there, and I couldn't help their racial feelings. A former bishop, who had given his life to Africa used to say "Always be just, never be kind", a truly shocking maxim. I suppose what he meant was "Always be fair, but don't be soft", but that was not how it sounded.

One day I went further afield than usual, visiting not only the familiar camps but following up abortive reports from new villages until at last the sun was down and I was still a long way from home. I pushed on through the growing darkness and at last reached a small mission in the bush, still some way short of the main road. I found an African deacon, the Revd. Gerard Sonje, in charge of the mission who gave me a kind welcome: he sat me in a deck chair and his wife made tea. Then their small son Silvester (now a very senior Medical Assistant) emerged from the kitchen bearing a bowl full of hard-boiled eggs—nothing else. I had been out since morning, and had eaten nothing but a few sandwiches at mid-day, it was now about 8 p.m. and I was thankful indeed for those eggs. We then went on together to the main road, and found Dr. Taylor out searching for me with the ambulance.

The epidemic eventually came to an end, and Dr. Taylor continued my introduction to the district. Then, rather less than six months after my arrival, she departed on a much-needed leave, and I was left on my own. For the next six months I was always on the move. I had to keep returning to Masasi, as I had been given the job of building a new outpatient block for the hospital. I knew nothing about building, but it appeared that the rest of the staff knew less, so I was told to do it. What emerged was a large building in sun-dried brick, with a stone floor and thatched roof. I learnt much in the process, chiefly about what to avoid another time, but the building stood and was still standing twenty-five years later, although it has gone now. My foreman was the senior dresser, Che Vincent Malunda, who had no more qualifications than I for building, but he knew about timber—which trees were ant-proof and where they could be found—and he knew how to get the best out of the workmen. Malunda was no longer young, but he was very active. His education had not gone far enough for him to acquire any recognised qualification, but what he lacked in that way was amply compensated for by experience, common sense and a shrewd judgement of people, especially patients. In his spare time he ran a small market garden, and he succeeded in growing potatoes where everyone said it was impossible. He was a tower of strength, with a great sense of humour. His brow was often furrowed with a concentration on one of a dozen problems but his kindly eyes twinkled behind his spectacles.

Meanwhile I was been called constantly from station to station, especially shuttling between Lulindi and Masasi sometimes by car, sometimes on foot or by bicycle, until I knew every hole in the road and almost every stick and stone. One evening I was called to Lulindi for two men who had been mauled by two different crocodiles. To save time I set out by bicycle. It did save time, but three hours' bicycling in the dark, through sand and into a head-wind, was far more tiring than seven hours' walking would have been. I arrived exhausted at about 9 p.m. Both patients were in a bad way: they had been carried in from many miles away, and one had already been lying on the river bank for some days before that. One had had an arm torn off, and the crocodile had also bitten right into his chest, piercing the lung. He was already in a desperate state, and died in the night. The other had had a leg mangled, the knee joint so twisted that it had burst wide open. I amputated his leg, but he had already been in that state for too long. Severe infection had set in—we had no penicillin in those days—and he too died soon after. Even before he was dead I had to return hastily to Masasi where more trouble was waiting.

Sometimes I was able to arrive in time to do some good, but often the distance the patient had to be brought, added to the time taken to bring me the news and then for me to get there, made the issue hopeless. Once at Lulindi I received a call to Masasi for a road-mender who had been trampled by an elephant, but on that occasion a messenger actually overtook the first to stop me from making a useless journey. From the description of his injuries it was clear that he could not possibly have lived.

These wild-beast accidents were the chief cause of serious injuries, and were always heavily infected. Crocodiles were the worst, owing to the size of their jaws and habit of snapping repeatedly at a man until he was lacerated from head to foot. A big one could bite a man in half—and then swallow one half. On one occasion two crocodiles were shot, after a fatal accident, and half the victim was found in each. But other accidents were from lion, leopard, hippopotamus, wild boar, buffalo, baboon, hyena and even the little bushbuck. I have known one cornered bushbuck disembowel a man, and two others break legs by butting. These accidents still happen, but with the coming of antibiotics their effects have become far less serious and many now live who in those days would have died.

Among the animals I have mentioned, the hippopotamus is one of the most dangerous, partly because of its size but even more because of its unpredictable behaviour. Although a strict vegetarian it will attack and bite savagely for no obvious reason, and in spite of its bulk it has a remarkable turn of speed on dry land. It spends all day lying inert in the water, only its eyes and nostrils above the surface (sometimes it even lies on the bottom for long periods without breathing at all) but at night it comes ashore and roams around consuming a vast quantity of greenery.

It is when a lone bull-hippo comes ashore by day that it becomes most dangerous. One, having wandered some twenty miles from the river, pursued a poor old man and trampled him to death for no reason at all. Another attacked a canoe, and having tipped the occupants into the river bit one of them right through the femur. The victim was carried to hospital at Newala, and eventually recovered. The Archdeacon of Luatala was also attacked by an angry hippo when in a canoe, but with great presence of mind opened and shut his umbrella in its face, and it went away.

Later, when I was at Mnero another hippo wandered some twenty miles from the river and, finding a small field of rice, proceeded to clear it up as already described. It then found and cleared a second field, but half-way through the third became so distended that it could eat no more, and lay down to sleep heavily. In this condition it was found by the villagers, who finding they had lost nearly all their rice came hot-foot to the Mission to ask for vengeance on the marauder. The Father Superior, a keen hunter, immediately set out with his rifle and arrived just as the hippo was waking up. It stood up suddenly and was about to charge, but too late. All the men of Mnero streamed out and cut up the hippo and there was meat for all. My students went out too, and won a good share. One of them, however said he could not eat any, as his family had a taboo against hippo. Later he received a letter from home saying that it was all right and that he could eat hippo, but by then the meat was finished. In the monastery we ate the tongue and the heart, and I have never tasted such tender and delicious meat.

In a country where there was no machinery and cars were scarce, other types of accident were rare. Apart from those caused by wild beasts, the commonest were hunting accidents—a home-made gun blowing up, or a hunter accidentally speared or shot by his companion; also, the results of beer fights. The people in those parts never fought sober, being too afraid of the endless repercussions in the village; but once this natural caution had been allayed by alcohol they were capable of inflicting serious injuries. One August Bank Holiday, I was enjoying some relaxation at Masasi when a message came that a badly injured man was being carried to Lulindi from a place thirty miles the other way. His nephew had borne a grudge against him for a long time, and the previous night, after a good deal of beer, went to his uncle's house and called him out; as soon as the uncle appeared he cracked him smartly over the head with an axe-haft. Dr. Taylor and I set off together by car, and were able to reach Lulindi before the patient, who was slowly being carried on a bed. We made some preparations, but when he arrived he had such a severe degree of cerebral compression that except for his pulse he appeared lifeless; his breathing was so slow that each breath appeared to be his last.

Unfortunately the primitive operating theatre had collapsed without warning so we could only operate in the little laboratory, where there was barely room to move. It was just a thatched hut, ten feet square, with unglazed windows and no running water. For light we had an electric torch and some hurricane lamps and for diathermy I used a silver probe heated red-hot in a spirit lamp. So utterly senseless was the patient that I was able to work without anaesthetic, but after I had removed some bone and a large blood-clot he began to recover so rapidly that he had to be held down while I sewed him up. The nephew was lucky to save his neck.

We treated a large number of knife wounds, not from fighting but from carelessness, owing to the custom of allowing small children to play freely with knives, and also from the usual method of carrying a naked knife tucked into the top of one's loincloth. On my first morning at Masasi a small girl was brought in who had fallen in a pit while playing with a knife. It had pierced her chest, and she had a large haemothorax, but the parents refused any operation and took her away. Another child was sent to herd goats, and getting bored tried to ride a large billy goat. The goat promptly threw him, and the knife in his loincloth pierced his loin. Luckily no serious harm was done, although the wound was deep.

A curious injury was sustained by an elderly and highly

respected teacher who had an evening out and was returning home in the dark. Having had too much to drink he literally fell by the wayside, and slept heavily, emitting loud snores. A young teacher from another village passing along the road heard this alarming noise and thought it must be a leopard, as leopards make a loud snoring noise at times. It was pitch dark, but he "drew his bow at a venture" in the direction of the snoring and planted an arrow in the old teacher's backside. Next morning the teacher came to hospital in considerable pain and greatly embarrassed, to have the wound dressed. The story had already spread far and wide.

Before I had been long on my own I had my first personal experience of amoebic dysentery. It took me suddenly one morning at Newala, but I was needed at Luatal, twenty miles away, so off I had to go. At Luatala I somehow survived a busy morning's work, including two operations, and then headed for Lulindi where there was more trouble waiting. It was evening before I reached Masasi, and as I stepped out of the ambulance a man emerged from the darkness with a letter. It was from Namasakata, 130 miles away, to say that the Sister in charge was down with sleeping-sickness. So I left again with the dawn and reached Namasakata in the afternoon. The Sister's fever had been taken in time, and treatment already begun, so after I had seen her I was able at last to retire to bed to receive some treatment for my dysentery. This unpleasant complaint was causing a lot of trouble among the staff at that time, and a few months later I had it again. The treatment tended then to be worse than the disease, but eventually I seemed to have acquired an adequate resistance to it, and could count one obstacle less.

Another personal problem was malaria. In those days the only prophylactic was quinine—five grains daily—which had only a very partial action. In spite of taking it with the utmost regularity I nevertheless had thirteen attacks of malaria in my first two years. Some were severe, including one which laid me up for a week and another which started at lunchtime; I shivered so much that I could hardly eat. My companions were engaged in an interminable discussion on the Swahili language, and completely ignored my condition. When at last they got up, one of them, also a doctor, said: "Now I'll take your temperature." It was 104.5 degrees, and I was quickly taken off to hospital. Over the years I gradually came to terms with the disease. We now have more effective prophylactics, but the old enemy is still active, albeit on a mild scale.

From early days I got used to walking from the forest at night, usually with companions, but sometimes with only a solitary porter or else completely alone with only my stick and my hurricane lamp for company. The object of these walks was to avoid the intolerable heat of the day, so for a twenty-four-mile journey I would start no later than 3 a.m. in order to arrive by ten o'clock before the worst of the heat. As these journeys were usually during the rains, when roads were closed to cars, it was always hot, even at night, and the darkness lent an extra oppressiveness to the heat as one plodded on and on along the narrow path, one eye open for snakes or a column of biting ants in the way, the other looking ahead at the grotesque shadows cast by the trees in the light of a hurricane lamp. Always there was the endless chorus of frogs, louder by the streams but always respectfully silenced as one passed and then opening up again behind. Every few miles one would meet a stream to be forded, the water tepid, the swirling sand entering one's shoes. The first streaks of dawn were always an immense relief, not only lightening the oppression of the darkness but also bringing a sharp and welcome drop in temperature with the formation of mist over the grass. One night at Masasi I was working late writing a report, and having planned to set out for Lulindi at 3 a.m. I thought it was pointless to go to bed; I would just work on. I did so, and at three o'clock picked up my stick and lamp and set out. I still felt quite fresh, but after the first hour I became so sleepy that I just could not continue. I sat down in the forest with my back against a tree for a short rest and immediately fell asleep. It was a lovely sleep, but when I woke with a jerk the dawn was breaking and I had lost nearly two hours of precious walking time. Dismayed I hurried on, but was hopelessly late. The day became hotter and hotter, and by 11 a.m. I was still far from home and sweltering in the heat. Again I sat under a tree, not to sleep but from sheer exhaustion. Then sweating and dizzy I plodded on, my steps becoming slower, the sand heavier and the sun ever hotter. At about noon I dragged myself into Lulindi, determined never to walk again. at night without having slept already.

Occasionally night-walks were undertaken somewhat unintentionally due to setting out on a day-time walk too late in the afternoon after a long day's work. Once, going to visit a dispensary, I was benighted with about five miles still to go. The path was through high forest; I had one of the Scouts (see Chapter XI) as a companion and no lamp. Fortunately, the path was straight, having once been cleared for wheeled traffic; it was now quite overgrown, but the gap in the trees remained, and could just be seen against the night sky as I kept looking up while feeling the path with my feet. There was no moon and in pitch darkness we just pushed on and on, until at last a little light appeared some way ahead. It was a lamp in the window of a lonely missionary, and we were glad to sleep there and finish our journey in the early morning.

6

Into the Wilderness

One morning at Masasi I saw an English woman dressed in a blue smock with a wide hat, and carrying a spear, walking into the hospital. They said she was a teacher from Lukwika. "Where is that?" I asked. "Three days into the wilderness" she replied. I was intrigued and the more I heard of Lukwika the more curious I was to go there. The place had a bad reputation: it was almost inaccessible except on foot, and atrociously hot; lions walked through the Mission and picked up anyone lying about; several missionaries had become unhinged in their minds after a prolonged stay and others had been evacuated sick, one at least in a dying condition. There was frequent famine, and a steadily dwindling and diseased population.

At last I had a chance to go there, accompanying Dr. Taylor on one of her visits. It was now the dry season and we were able to go in her indestructible "B-Model" Ford, but even so the road was appalling, bridges hardly existed and the fifty-six miles took us all day, so that we arrived dirty, hot and tired as the sun was setting. At least I learnt the road, and so was prepared when later, during the rains and in Dr. Taylor's absence on leave, I received an emergency call there.

This time there was no question of motoring, but I found the idea of a three days' walk through hot, rough country hard to face, so I borrowed a bicycle. It was an old but sound ladies' model. It also had a basket strapped to the handle-bars, into which I crammed my essential needs. As the morning Angelus began to ring at 6 a.m., I pedalled off down the hill from Masasi and into the wilderness. At first I made quite good progress, following a well-used and still passable motor-road for the first eight miles. Then I turned off on to the Lukwika road proper, and abruptly conditions became worse. At first there were alternations of sand and mud, with plenty of holes and a good deal of long grass, but after Kawela the sand began to give place to stones and rocks, and the mud to stretches of water. Meanwhile the sun was going up and up, and the heat was increasing. Presently in a low lying stretch I came to a real "Slough of Despond". The road simply disappeared into a wide stretch of soft black mud and standing water, which for good measure and to show what they thought of the road, the local people had planted with rice. A foot-track remained through the middle, but at every step I and the bicycle sank a foot deep into the stinking black mud. Riding was out of the question, and even pushing it was soon impossible. I had to hoist it on my shoulder, feeling like the man and his son who decided to carry their ass. In the slough it was hotter than ever, flies and insects buzzed, and the frogs mocked me. At last I was through, and began to ride again, the wheels spraying mud. Towards midday I reached the fork of the old and new roads, and realised I had made good time. The new road was the better, but I took the old one, as I wanted to stop at the Mission rest-house at Nauru, which the new road would by-pass. I soon reached it, and as it was now very hot indeed I was glad of a rest in the shade.

The rest-house was the usual mud hut with grass thatch, containing a bare string bed and a table and chair. I ate my sandwich lunch and stretched out on the bed for a couple of hours. While I slept it rained heavily, and when I set out again the sun was less fierce. However, the road now deteriorated even more. This, being the old road, had not been repaired for several years, and as it crossed several deep and steep gullies and streams, it was totally broken up. I clambered down the gullies and crawled up the other side dragging the bicycle with its precious basket. All the earth of the road had long been washed away, and only rocks and stones were left. I scrambled and hauled, falling into holes and sweating up hills. The detour of the old road was supposed to be only two miles, but it seemed endless, and I was getting more and more tired and disheartened. Where the road was not actually washed away it was overgrown with grass and dense weeds and thorns.

At last, when I was coming to the end of my tether, I regained the new road, with some fear that I might get benighted. The road improved for a bit, but then I reached a stream which was swollen by the rain and I had to wade through thigh-deep, dragging the bicycle as best I could. Then I met the tsetse flies, which are very difficult to beat off when one is riding a bicycle. They bite hard, and cause furious itching. There was plenty more mud and water and several streams, but at last, sometime after 5 p.m. I passed the village of Chungu, about seven miles short of Lukwika, and at last the road improved. It was still all grassed over, but walking feet had worn a single narrow track, and this was smooth sand which had been packed down by the rain and made into a firm cycling surface. And, most welcome of all, the road began a slight but steady downhill run which was not noticeable when we were motoring but which, I now joyfully realised, would carry me almost to Lukwika. I began to speed along, with an enormous sense of relief. There was no more habitation, just the forest, dense and dark and overgrown with the rains, the wet grass swishing by, puddles splashing, but myself sailing always on and down. It seemed almost too good to be true, as I went faster and faster with less and less effort. Then suddenly on my right I saw through the trees a great rock. I could hardly believe it, but it must be the look-out rock from which one could look out over the forest and the Mission and all the country around. I nearly shouted for joy, and in another moment I was bumping down the steep rough approach to the sandy crossing of the last river. I dragged the bike up the other bank, and set out to ride the last half-mile through the mud-flats and the high grass. This was the point from which motorists always tooted their horn to announce their coming, so I rang my bell as hard as I could, but I doubt if anyone heard. A few minutes later I was pedalling up the short steep stony approach to the Mission with my last bit of strength. As I rode in, the evening Angelus began to ring: it was 6 p.m., exactly twelve hours since I had left Masasi. I was covered with mud and sweat, and my legs hardly seemed to belong to me, but I had arrived.

I dealt with the emergency forthwith, and after some food went to sleep. By next morning I was in the throes of acute dysentery again, so spent an enforced ten days at Lukwika being treated, and while convalescing was able to look at the place more closely. It was certainly remote. As I have said, the population was dwindling, and from the Mission, on its little hill, no single habitation could be seen, only the forest stretching endlessly and utterly silent. You watched the road for someone approaching, but saw nothing. You listened for any sound, but only heard the distant cry of a lone bird and the rustle of a breeze in the dry grass, then silence again. Always the sun beat down and the heat shimmered off the quartz gravel that covered the hill.

There was little work to do in the hospital, as there were so few people, so as soon as I was fit I set out for home. Because of the debilitating effects of dysentery treatment, as then practised, I decided not to try cycling again but to go on foot, and to cut across country directly to Lulindi, which was about sixty miles. I also began by being carried for alternate hours in a hammock, but by the second day I had had enough of its discomfort (it sounds good but is anything but) and decided it was better to walk all the time. The road back was the same as far as Nauru where I had rested on the way out, but then the five of us (I was accompanied by the two men with the hammock, a cook and a porter with provisions) left the so-called road and cut straight through the forest on a narrow path. I had intended to sleep at Nauru, but we had arrived early and I felt fitter than I expected, so after a meal we went on. It was dark when we reached Minje, where we found an old man grilling leopard-meat while the skin was stretched out to dry. I had never heard of anyone eating leopard, but maybe all he was doing was preparing "medicine" in order to bewitch someone. Minje was a very small village deep in the forest and utterly lonely in the wet darkness. There was a tiny mission rest-hut, half filled by an enormous anthill, but I squeezed in and was able to sleep there.

Next morning we started early, and continued through the forest. After an hour or two we could hear the roaring of water and knew we were approaching the Mbangala river. For a long time we were walking near it but could see nothing through the high grass. Then at last we came suddenly on the bank, and saw a great swirling down between huge rocks with a magnificent mountain towering over it. There had been plenty of rain, and the river was in good spate, but it looked as if we could cross. We chose a likely spot where the path came down to the water's edge, and began fording. The current was strong and progress was necessarily slow. By the middle the water was nearly to our hips and pressing strongly. However, it got no deeper and eventually we were safely across, the box of provisions balanced on the head of the porter.

Beyond the river there was a long stretch through tall grass, again close to the invisible torrent, the heat now very oppressive, and strange and sickening smells rising from the rank vegetation. At last we got out of the valley and climbed a little into the forest again, where it was not so hot. We eventually came to Njawara, and then dropping into another valley forded the Miesi, another fast river swirling with suspended mud, but that day not more than knee deep. After Miesi we climbed a little and by midday had reached Lipumburu, where we were glad to rest. There was a small mission there, and after I had sat down and emptied the water from my shoes, the wife of the old African priest-in-charge, the late Revd. Obed Y. Kasembe, brought me tea and half a pumpkin, boiled whole and served hot. I had never before met pumpkin prepared like that, but after eating it all, I decided I never again wanted pumpkin done in any other way. Chopping, mashing, sieving, and so on simply destroy what little taste it has, nor is this remedied by the addition of caraway seeds!

I had a long talk with the old priest, from whom I learnt much of the history of the Mission and the activities of his people. With his acute intellect and sly sense of humour, he was very independent and something of an embarrassment to the Bishop.

We left at 3 a.m. next day for the twenty-four miles to Lulindi, and were past Mtojo before the dawn, and then on to Lukondesi as the sun came up behind the hill of Huwe. After that it was familiar country, through the fields and woods, fording the Mwiti river, and coming safely home to Lulindi, sweating but content, by 11 a.m. I now felt fit again and the dysentery was a thing of the past. I sat on my verandah and drank five mugs of black tea. Then I had a bath and picked up the threads of my work again. I had of course left the bicycle to find its own way home, but it soon turned up safe.

Some time later I heard of a horrible tragedy at Lukwika. A young English nurse had gone to the hospital store to draw methylated spirit from a drum. Having filled her bottle she attempted to seal the drum with molten wax from a lighted candle. Of course the vapour of the spirit ignited and the drum exploded. The nurse was burnt to death, and the store totally destroyed with a whole year's supply of drugs and equipment. All the buildings were grass-thatched and the fire leapt from roof to roof destroying several more of them. It seems incredible that any skilled worker should have been so foolish, and yet a few months later this folly was precisely repeated at Mikindani. On this occasion the building was a stone one, so only the stores were destroyed. The perpetrator was a very senior dresser, who was himself only slightly burnt, but his friend the teacher, standing ten yards away, was hit by a great tongue of flame which burnt his legs. He eventually recovered from his burns, but at the time he had been suffering from severe hookworm infestation, and the burning precipated an acute state of vitamin deficiency, as a result of which he developed bilateral cataract and rapidly became completely blind. He retired to his village in the bush, where he soon died of pneumonia.

Lukwika was eventually closed down and evacuated. The lions were left in possession and no-one was sorry. But the few old hands who were still alive then must have felt sad, if they heard of it, for all the heroic work that was once done and forgotten in the unforgiving forest.

Anyone living in Africa is sometimes asked if he has met many lions: one meets them occasionally, though normally they go their way and I go mine. One came on to my verandah one night and made a great noise worrying a bone, but I shone a light at it through the window and shouted, and it bounded off. I have met others crossing the road at night, caught momentarily in the beam of the headlights.

The lion is not respected here as the King of the Beasts, but is regarded rather as a vulgar nuisance which may at any time become a menace. An African friend said "We cannot admire the lion: you see, we are his food"—a chilling thought. Until a lion has acquired the habit of man-eating, however, he is an indolent and often cowardly creature, who can be seen off even by a determined pack of dogs, wild or even domestic.

A missionary met two men on a forest path, carrying a big piece of meat on a pole. Supposing they had been hunting, he congratulated them on their good luck. They replied that they had found a lion eating it, but they had beaten the lion and taken it away from him. The same missionary, on another journey through the forest, in the half-light of early morning, saw what he took to be a tree-stump beside the path, then suddenly realised that it was a sitting lion. "Oh dear", he said to the porter, "what shall we do?" "You are always telling us to trust in God," replied the porter, "Why not try it now?" So they shouted loudly, and the lion went off.

Another missionary had trouble with his jeep, and finally came to a stop just at the place where I had met two huge lions a few nights before. Not knowing this, he got out, opened the bonnet and began tinkering with the distributor. Having finished the repair he stood up to stretch his back and looked straight into the face of a large lion which sat quietly watching from the other side of the engine. He simply leaped into the jeep and left at full speed.

A man-eater, however, is very different, and when one starts on this career, there is often a long toll of deaths before it is killed. The mother of one of my students was eaten by a lion, and after a time his father set off to look for a new wife, and on the way he was caught and eaten too. My student told this to me in a completely matter-of-fact way: it was only too common where he came from.

Tandahimba (which means "lion-lake") had man-eaters from time to time. One day when a pair of them was about, a man was returning home at dusk, and was nearly at his house when he suddenly saw a lion sitting very quietly among the cassava bushes only a few yards away, watching him. Seeing no escape whatever, he dropped to his knees and made the sign of the cross. Then, in a movement of utter helplessness, he simply flopped back on his heels. As he did so, something brushed past his face—it was the lioness, who as usual was doing the hunting while her lord and master sat watching. She had made her spring from some yards away, unseen by her intended victim, and was in mid-air when his sudden drop backwards spoilt her aim by inches, and she crashed harmlessly into the bushes. She was so put off that both lions bounded away, while the man scrambled into his house.

My last incident concerns a man who had been out drinking, and when the beer was all finished he set out for home. As it was completely dark he took a burning brand with him to light his way, and as the world seemed to be turning over and over he found it safer to proceed on hands and knees. After crawling some way like this along the narrow path to his home, he came to a place where the path narrowed still more between two posts. He stopped, puzzled. Even in his fuddled condition he was sure there had been no posts in the path when he left home. He blew on his brand to light up the posts, and following them upwards, he found that they merged in a great hairy chest, and above that was the face of a huge lion. Suddenly sobered, he thrust the burning brand into the lion's mouth and fled. Believe this last story or not—I have recounted it as it was told to me.

7

Tropical Surgery and Traditional Medicine

After Dr. Taylor's return in 1936 I was able to settle at Lulindi and develop the hospital there. I was also responsible for the hospitals at Newala and Luatala and their subsidiary dispensaries, so I was still often on the move. I tried to divide my time fairly between the different stations, but the only result of this was that they all felt equally hurt and each reproached me in turn with giving all my attention to the other stations.

On one occasion I was passing Luatala on my way home from an expedition, and looked in to see if all was well. The Sister in charge of the dispensary at that time had the aim in life of maintaining the utmost calm even when people were dying all around her. Calm is good, but she carried it rather far, and I had got to know her, so when she said that all was quiet, and "there is only old Mariamŭ but she is dying of cancer, you can't do anything for her", I decided I would go and see for myself.

From one look at poor Mariamu, it was clear that she was dying, but not of cancer. She had a strangulated hernia of the pelvic colon of unknown duration, and was already cold, pulseless and hardly conscious. Saying little to the Sister (after all, nurses are not supposed to diagnose) I got the old lady into the tiny mud hut called the "operating theatre" as fast as possible, injected some local anaesthetic (all she could stand) and made a rapid caecostomy. Although I worked fast, it was not fast enough to avoid a lump of dirty grass from the thatch falling right on to the exposed caecum. However, I washed it off and no harm was done.

As there was nothing more I could do (at Luatala we had no intravenous solutions or blood and few drugs) I went for some supper. Before going to bed I enquired after the patient, and was surprised and gratified to be told that she was talking volubly and asking for tea. A week later I was able to transfer her by ambulance to Lulindi and do some more extensive surgery. As a girl she had survived the terrible disease known as *cancrum oris*, in those days normally a killer, so she was obviously tough. She lived happily for long afterwards.

On another visit to Luatala I was suddenly faced by a party of men carrying the dead bodies of two old women with a letter from the District Commissioner demanding a post-mortem. Enquiry elicited the following story. The two old women had been attacked and battered to death by a young madman, who said afterwards that he had a message from God to kill all the women in his village; the young ones had all run too fast and escaped. The two bodies had been buried in defiance of the D.C.'s order for an inquest, but as the village was remote, it was three weeks before the D.C. learned that his order had been ignored. He then said he "would teach the village headman a lesson", and ordered the bodies to be exhumed and transported to the nearest doctor for post-mortem. Thus on one of the hottest days in the year these two liquefying corpses of three weeks' incubation, which had been carried on poles for some forty miles under the tropical sun, were dumped at my feet. To make matters worse, it was about 2 p.m. on a fast-day, so I had eaten nothing since the day before. I duly did the post-mortems in a small hut (I will not attempt to describe them) and made sure of collecting my hard-earned fee, but I felt the "lesson" intended for the headman had been effectively passed on to me.

The first essential at Lulindi was to build a proper operating theatre, and this I took in hand at once. Costs were then absurdly low, and the completed building of theatre and three anterooms cost less than £100.

For the building I used the experience gained at Masasi, and evolved a simple style which proved satisfactory over the years. Building meant beginning from scratch. Earth had to be dug and bricks made. Trees had to be cut in the forest and sawn up by hand to make boards. For beams we used hardwood trees in the round, simply trimming off the soft outer wood. Stone for the floors had to be carted from a nearby hill in the ambulance. It was not necessary to quarry it but trimming the blocks to the correct shape made a lot of work. There were few local Africans who had any experience of stonework or bricklaying, but we managed to import some from Masasi and Ndanda. Most of these were not very skilful and needed constant supervision. In particular they were quite unable to follow a straight line, and in fact seemed to have no conception of what it meant. Later, however, after trying many so-called masons, I did find two or three who could do really good work unsupervised. Two of them built a large dispensary with no help from me except in marking out the foundations, and made an excellent job of it. These two took the leading part in the building of the wards for Lulindi Hospital (described later) and one of them, Sebastian, had the melancholy distinction of being the first patient to be admitted to his beautiful building, where he then died of inoperable cancer.

Owing to the expense of corrugated iron, I still used grass for thatching, on a framework of bamboo closely bound with a very strong bast from the forest. Thatch is not only picturesque, but also cool; however, there its advantages end. It gets blown about by whirlwinds, it leaks, it harbours rats, snakes and white ants, and always there is the danger of fire; with thatch this means the end of the house and everything in it. The original grass is cheap, but the work of thatching is not if one uses expert thatchers, without whom it will not last. Also the grass must be renewed every few years, so it is a recurring expense. Later, in disgust, I gave up thatch and began to make tiles (see Chapter XIV).

Lime could be got from local lime-burners at Masasi, if they could be stimulated to burn any—it was only a casual occupation for them. Otherwise it had to be brought from the coast, 100 miles away, as did cement and any simple fittings such as nails, bolts and hinges. Glass and any more elaborate fittings had to be ordered from Dar es Salaam—400 miles away.

The theatre proved very satisfactory in use, and the only subsequent addition that I found necessary was an extra sterilising room. We had no running water, but at least we had adequate lighting from inverted paraffin-vapour lamps of 800 candle-power. The first time they were lit at night people came running from all around to know what the blaze of light could be. It was just as well I had fitted shutters to frustrate the inquisitive during operations at night.

Surgery in those days was done under considerable difficulties. Besides the patient's natural fear of an operation there was the complication that any injury to an individual was in African eyes an injury to the family, and so before an operation could be done not only was the consent of the patient essential but also that of all his relatives. Even if the patient were willing, the obstinate refusal of some old man, or even more often some old woman, would often make it impossible to operate, and one had to watch the patient dying slowly of a condition that could easily have been relieved. On one occasion a damaged eye needed urgent removal to save the sight of the other. Everyone had agreed, when a message came from the Chief, Mwenye Che Matola II, then more than ninety years old: "The eye is not to be removed", and everything was at a standstill. I went to remonstrate with the Chief. He shook his head and in a senile whisper replied "Remove eye—die." Fortunately I was able to ask him whether he knew a certain European? Yes, he said, what of it? I explained that that man had only one eye, while the other was made of glass. He was astounded, but when the truth of this was confirmed by some of his people he said very well then, take it out.

Occasionally this collective responsibility had its uses. Once a woman refused an urgent operation, but her family decided she should have it, and ignoring her screams of protest they carried her bodily into the theatre and held her down until she was anaesthetised. Even when consent had been given our troubles were not over, for the whole family insisted on being present at the operation. This was mainly to make sure that bits of the patient were not taken away to be made into "medicine" for use in witchcraft.

Later I was able to reduce the family representation to two and then to one, who had to be properly garbed in cap and mask and sit quietly in a corner. In the end I inserted a special window, so that the relatives could sit in an ante-room and watch all that went on in the theatre. Nowadays few of them trouble to do so.

Gynaecology accounted for much of the surgery, increasingly so as the women's confidence was gained. One woman arrived with an enormous ovarian cyst, complicated by a well-advanced pregnancy. I wanted to remove the cyst, as I did not see how she could deliver a child while it was blocking the way. However, the patient refused firmly, saying she would have the child first and come back later for the operation. I never thought I should see her again but some months later, to my great surprise, she turned up, smiling happily and carrying a fine child in her arms. "You see", she said, "I have got my baby and now I have come back for the operation. I told you I would!" I removed the cyst and it was too big to go into a bucket. All the family came to marvel at it, and went home very pleased.

Another woman came from further away, beyond the Ruvuma, with a hard mass that felt like a fibroid uterus. I operated, but when I tried to deliver the uterus in the ordinary way, it jumped right out on the table. It was no uterus at all, but a very large solid fibroma of one ovary. This was very easy to remove, and I took it along later to show the patient. I thought she would be pleased, but she didn't even smile. She gave the tumour a very sour look, and said with real hatred in her voice, "Now I'm going home to find out who put that thing in my belly." She disappeared soon after without paying her modest bill (operations were only 1*s*. each in those days) and probably spent large sums to pin the tumour, by divination, on some wretched neighbour. The tumour may well have caused endless suspicion and maltreatment of quite innocent people, and it might have been better if I had never removed it.

Quite early on I treated a childless couple, and in due course they had a baby. I think the baby might well have arrived even without my treatment, but the word went round that I could get babies for sterile couples, and the reputation pursued me ever after, even from one hospital to another. One couple came all the way from Dar es Salaam, 400 miles away. It was really very embarrassing, as the treatment of infertility is no simple matter. It shows how a reputation sticks, when once acquired, regardless of performance. (I did have a few gratifying successes, but plenty of failures too).

When one is the only doctor (and I was single-handed for twenty-nine years in all) and doing much surgery, anaesthesia is a serious problem. I tackled this problem in various ways, making considerable use of local and regional anaesthesia, and teaching all my trained nurses to give ether. But for major operations I found it best to rely whenever possible on spinal anaesthesia. This had never been popular in Britain, and when I was a student had only been practised in a very haphazard way by a few anaesthetists, with highly unpredictable and sometimes even fatal results. However, by the time I came to Africa it was becoming established on a rational basis, although its use was still limited, and the introduction of heavy Nupercaine instead of the classical Stovaine made it both safer and far more effective. I followed and adapted the technique of Michael Nosworthy, and found I could obtain completely satisfactory, prolonged and safe anaesthesia up to the fifth rib. With a suitable sedative the patient sleeps peacefully and you have total relaxation of his muscles, reduced bleeding and peace in the theatre. With a capable nurse to watch the patient and take his blood-pressure regularly, the surgeon can concentrate on his work without keeping "one eye on the anaesthetic". However, one must have an exact technique and keep rigidly to the rules. With the slightest deviation, failure and even disaster are just round the corner.

I had not been long at Lulindi when I was called one day to Masasi, in Dr. Taylor's absence, to deal with a very bad compound leg fracture. The patient was in great pain, and as usual there was no skilled anaesthetist available, so I gave him a spinal anaesthetic. Both the patient and the hospital staff, who had not seen this "medicine" before, were amazed at the rapid and total relief of pain. The patient was pathetically grateful and talked as I worked on his leg. "I was only helping my neighbour", he said. "She is a poor widow, and was trying to cut down a tree by herself, so I went to help her and the tree fell on my leg." I did what I could for him, but his condition was bad. In those days at Masasi we had no antibiotics, no blood-transfusion, nor even any intravenous infusions—little in fact beyond morphia and hope. It was not enough, and he died. A hundred years earlier he would have had an immediate amputation, willy-nilly, which would probably have saved his life, but in the climate of opinion at Masasi in 1935 he would never have consented to losing his leg.

With modern anaesthetic facilities spinal anaesthesia is irrelevant and even troublesome, but in single-doctor bush hospitals it still enables patients to have effective and often life-saving treatment which would otherwise be impossible or at the very least, hazardous.

In those early days surgery accounted for the smaller part of the work, but this was to change remarkably with the years. Most of our work was with the common tropical diseases. I have already mentioned yaws, bilharzia and hookworm infestation. Commoner than any of these was malaria, which to some degree affected the entire population. The worst sufferers were the children, who had to acquire their relative immunity the hard way, by surviving attack after attack of fierce fever. Many did not survive. Often a child would be playing happily in the evening and be dead before morning, or would survive just long enough to be brought to hospital unconscious, limp and grey, beyond the help of any medicine. The mortality of infants and toddlers was heartbreaking and I would estimate that a majority of first children never grew up. Malaria tipped the balance against them.

Leprosy was also common, afflicting 30 per 1000 of the population, and amoebic dysentery was endemic. Relapsing fever and sleeping-sickness were uncommon, but turned up occasionally in patients from certain areas. Add to these scabies, eye infections, and ulcers of every sort and you have a general picture of our daily work. There were also of course many cases of non-tropical complaints such as pneumonia, meningitis and septic infections, and from time to time we had epidemics of measles and whooping-cough, both often fatal for small children.

What was most satisfying about dealing with the tropical diseases was that each had a specific remedy and if taken in time could be cured, even before the advent of modern antibiotics. Many of the commoner and less easily curable diseases of Europe, on the other hand, were rarely seen, such as high blood-pressure, peptic ulcer, organic heart disease, inflammations of the kidneys and gall-bladder, and diabetes. Appendicitis was also curiously rare, and the few cases seen were all mild. Contrary to popular belief, however, many varieties of cancer were seen.

The nearest dentist being fifty miles away, we had to pull a lot of teeth. At that time I had not yet pirated enough dental skill to give effective local anaesthetics, so we just pulled in cold blood. However, the local people quite expected it that way: if a tooth ached they wanted it out, and did not bother about anaesthesia. I had two out myself the same way, there being no other, at the able hands of one of the nurses or dressers. The dressers were better, as the nurses had not always the brute strength that is sometimes needed. Later I learned to give a mandibular block, and dental extractions became very popular.

Our patients came from as far as ten miles away, and would do the journey daily if necessary. Those who came prepared to stay in, might have come many days' walk. Many came down from the Makonde plateau, others from the Ruvuma river and from Mozambique beyond it. Some came even from the coast, 100 miles away. They brought their food with them, and one or more relatives to cook and care for them. Often the whole family came, and even brought their hens. Most members of the family had some complaint, and would take the opportunity to obtain some medicine. In those days they had to do much of their own nursing, as our trained staff was still small.

The patients brought their payment in kind, and by the end of a busy morning the outpatient verandah looked like a harvest festival. The food was quickly priced by a senior dresser, and afterwards stored to help feed indigent patients.

We received people of different tribes, and because many, especially the women, could not speak Swahili, I had to acquire at least the rudiments of three more languages.

Most patients had already tried a number of local remedies first, and some had even been to other hospitals, so the clinical picture was seldom uncomplicated. Some were merely suffering from poisonous herbal remedies.

Traditional or herbal remedies have no system of testing or

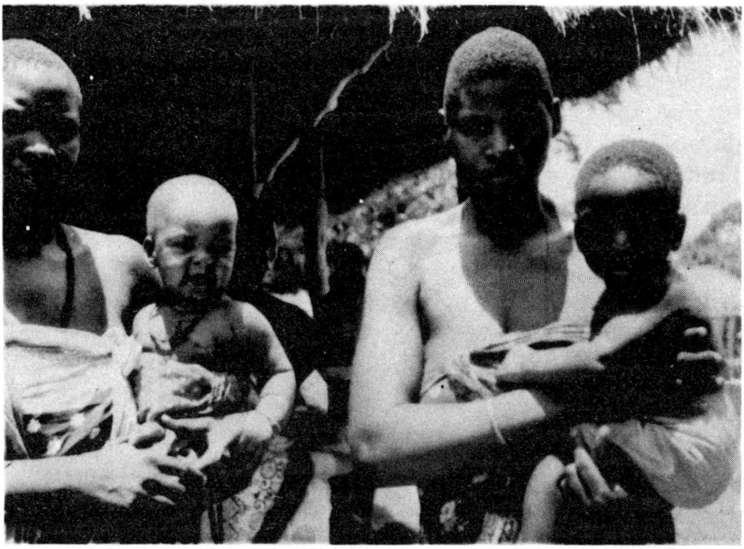

Children at Lulindi clinic

measurement, and are rarely given by a medicine-man without some form of charm or divination. Books have been written about them, and I shall not go deeply into the subject. It is enough to record that most of our patients had tried these local remedies before coming to the hospital (often the last resort), and that they cost far more than our modest fees. Because of the lack of measurement, children were often heavily over-dosed, and many were brought to hospital suffering from poisonous effects, rather than from any serious disease. Some of them died. However, there is no doubt that some of these medicines are valuable, and I was able to test and approve at least one. A child was brought with a large burn on one thigh, and I saw that the burn had been coated with a sticky substance. This was not unusual, as most burns had received some first-aid application, often lamp-oil or honey. In this case, however, the appearance was quite impressive, so instead of cleaning off the medicine I simply applied some dry gauze and bandaged it. After ten days I gently peeled off the gauze, and saw a perfectly clean, healed, area of skin. On enquiring I found that this application was latex from the bark of a tree called *mtomoni*. It obviously contained plenty of tannic acid, and was also a strong adhesive. These two constituents made a most effective coagulation-dressing, (this was long before tannic acid had come into disrepute) and I subsequently recommended *mtomoni* for burns in my first-aid instructions to the Scouts. These herbal medicines and their associated charms are used for many purposes besides illness, in fact for almost any of life's problems whether domestic, social, commercial, or anything else. A local chief had a grudge against an elderly deacon, so he secreted a packet of medicine in the roof of the deacon's house. Before long a whirlwind completely removed the thatch, but the deacon felt his enemy had been worsted, as the medicine in the roof was now exposed to public view, and the chief was thus put to public shame. In other words, loss of face is worse than loss of thatch.

At all our hospitals and dispensaries ulcers of the leg, both chronic and acute, were the biggest constant problem. These came daily in vast numbers and hideous in extent. The underlying causes were many, and included initial trauma, insect bites, yaws, leprosy, malnutrition and anaemia from many causes (but not varicose veins, which were unknown). The ulcers were often huge and deep, and lasted even for years. After fifteen years they were liable to develop cancer and the leg would have to be amputated. The acute ulcers (the exact cause of which is still a matter of dispute) were liable in sickly children to progress to the condition known as phagedena, with rapid destruction of skin, muscles and even bones, the smaller bones of the foot simply dropping out onto the dressing. These children often died. Even if they rallied and recovered it was with terrible scarring and deformities. So numerous were the ulcer cases that in every hospital it was necessary to have a special room, even a separate hut, set aside for treating them; to provide enough dressing material it was necessary to beg loads of worn-out sheets and shirts from friends in England, which could be torn up to make both dressings and bandages. Hospital gauze in the quantity required was beyond the purse of the Mission or the contributions which the patients could afford.

Where are these ulcers now? In a day's work at Kibosho, my last hospital (Chapter XIX), we might see one ulcer, possibly two. Penicillin, shoes, trousers, better diet, the disappearance of yaws and the effective treatment of leprosy have dealt a death blow to the ulcer. This is probably the biggest and most striking single change that has come about in recent years in the practice of tropical medicine.

I did little domiciliary medicine, as the conditions were so unfavourable, and anyhow the lack of facilities for nursing usually made it necessary to insist on the patient being brought into hospital before any treatment could be given. However, I did occasionally pay a visit, either to increase confidence where there was some reluctance to come to hospital, or to show practical sympathy where the family was in distress. I had a light canvas visiting bag which could be slung over my shoulder or strapped to the back of my bicycle, and so equipped I would follow the narrow paths through the forest and the fields of millet or beans to the sick man's hamlet. There was no door-bell or even knocker. In any case it is difficult to knock on a door made of millet stalks or bamboos. One just calls out the untranslatable '*Hodi*' at the door and awaits the welcoming reply of '*Hodini*' (literally '*hodi* to you') or '*Karibu*' ('Draw near'). Only then (and saying '*Hodi*' again for safety and politeness) can one go in. The average hut then had no windows, and one made a sudden transition from brilliant sunlight to darkness, usually made worse by a smoking fire, and walls and a roof blackened all over by soot. I just had to stand waiting till my eyes had adapted themselves. Presently I could just make out the interior—I was often guided to the bed by the patient's groans. The first thing then was to give the patient '*Pole!*', the universal expression of sympathy, literally 'Gently!' (i.e. 'take it easy') but meaning more 'I am sorry for your trouble', as the Irish say. Then I could begin my questioning, and such examination as was possible in the darkness. Occasionally I would leave some medicine, but more often it was necessary to organise the transfer of the patient to hospital in a hammock or on an upturned bed. The beds were made only of light wooden poles, laced across with palm leaf strings, so they were light to carry. A longer pole was lashed with more palm-leaf rope between the upturned legs, and supported on two men's shoulders.

Sometimes, in spite of all my persuasion and expressions of sympathy, the patient, or his family, refused absolutely to come in. One such case was a woman with tetanus. As in those days tetanus patients usually died, I was worried at her refusing the small chance offered by hospitalisation, and went away warning her relatives of the worst. "I shall stay here, and get better at home", she said—and she did.

I had barely settled at Lulindi when the tribal initiation rites began. These occurred about every third year, and involved the segregation of all the uninitiated boys and girls into secret camps. The boys were kept in the forest, where they were first circumcised, and then taught tribal traditions and good manners until they were healed. Then they were brought back to the village dressed in new clothes with huge rejoicing and much dancing and drinking. The circumcisions were carried out in completely primitive and barbaric fashion, the boys lying in the dust surrounded by a howling, yelling mob, while fierce drumming drowned their cries. Naturally there was always much trouble afterwards, from septic wounds, haemorrhage, and other complications, and the idea had got about that it was a good thing to ask the doctor and his assistants to come along and apply some European dressings to the wounds. I consequently attended a number of these circumcisions, but found the conditions utterly impossible for applying any useful treatment, owing to the indescribable dirt and confusion that prevailed. The problem was made more difficult by the fact that the Mission had given its blessing to these ceremonies, in an expurgated form, and the mission hospital was expected to give full support. This encouragement also increased the popularity of the rites, at a time when in other areas they were rapidly dying out.

In that year and the next five years I examined and treated 1,000 boys in these initiation camps, and with the loyal cooperation of my dressers tried every means we could devise to bring order out of chaos and to establish some sort of antiseptic regime. We even undertook circumcisions ourselves where the people would agree. But the conditions were utterly impossible, and in the end I could only urge that all boys should be brought to hospital for circumcision. After the five years I embodied my experiences and recommendations in a careful report, which I presented to the Bishop. His only comment was that when I had been in the Mission rather longer I might see things differently. I still have a copy of that report, and even now, after more than thirty years, would not alter a word of it.

8
Training Nurses

It soon became clear that our greatest need was a properly trained African staff. The European staff were few, and fewer stayed the course. It was obvious that for any promising future, African doctors and nurses were needed who could eventually replace us completely. The Mission had made a start in training young men as 'Dispensers' (later known as Medical Assistants) at Minaki near Dar es Salaam, but no trainee who had finished the course had yet reached the Masasi diocese. Some of our dressers were good and reliable, but their training had been irregular and fortuitous, and they had only the most elementary educational background. At Lulindi the two juniors, John and Dominic, were bright boys, quite young, with whom I hoped rather more might be achieved. They were keen and alert and took a real interest in their work, but all too soon John became entangled with a schoolgirl and had to leave. Dominic, who was a Makonde, generally but mistakenly regarded as a backward tribe, was always laughing and was everybody's friend. He became particularly friendly with a boy patient who was having treatment for a contracted knee-joint, caused by an attack of meningitis. When Dominic himself had to go into hospital for a minor ailment, he shared a hut with his friend. No one suspected that this boy was still a carrier of the disease, until a few days later I was horrified to find Dominic with a headache and a stiff neck. Sulphonamides had not then reached us in the bush, and there was nothing we could do to prevent him from getting rapidly worse. Still cheerful, and remarkably conscious almost to the end, he developed bulbar paralysis and died on the critical fifth day. (In pre-antibiotic days, it was said that a patient with meningitis who survived the fifth day of disease would usually recover).

African doctors were for us still out of the question. We had no one approaching the necessary education. But nurses were as much needed, and here we could make a start, although suitably educated girls were few. The idea of trained female nurses was received on most sides with amazement and even disapproval. It had never been done and was an impossible project. Our first student-nurse, Judith Ligunda, at Luatala, did not last long, for reasons not connected with her work, but later she joined Government service and eventually became a Matron in the National Service. Then at Lulindi Miss Bell, who shared my views on the urgency of proper training, made a start with two more. Neither of these ever finished the course, but before they left, others had joined, and a solid foundation had been laid which was eventually to produce excellent results. Our first nurse to complete the course (now Mrs. Thekla Mchauru, she was also the first Tanganyikan woman to qualify as a teacher) qualified in 1940, the first Tanganyikan woman to become a registered nurse. This was actually the first nursing school in Tanganyika to obtain official recognition and at that time even Government had not begun to train nurses. (Magila Hospital had been training nurses rather longer, but had not yet sought official recognition, so their nurses could not yet be registered.)

One of the biggest obstacles to training nurses or medical assistants was that heads of schools held on to all their brightest pupils and channelled them into teacher-training, under the mistaken impression that teaching was the only respectable profession. This idea died hard, and for years restricted us almost entirely to those who failed to be thus selected for teacher-training. One of our teachers once urged me to accept a boy for training. She was praising his character so much, and was so insistent that I should accept him that I could not help asking innocently why he should not become a teacher. She exclaimed, "You see, he hasn't a brain in his head!"

By this time I had completed my probationary two years and was due for six months' leave. When the time came I was laid up with a very persistent abscess of one leg, and could only move on crutches. The roads were closed again by the rains, and I was faced with the necessity of a hundred-mile walk to the coast. The only way was to be carried in a hammock. So this was arranged, and we set out one morning at 2 a.m. Carrying a man in a hammock is hard work for the carriers, and is also a remarkably uncomfortable mode of transport for the passenger. My feet were higher than my head, and I went bump, bump, bump with every step till I felt quite sick. Soon we were climbing the escarpment of the Makonde plateau, and as it became steeper I was simply dragged up, two men pushing the hammock-pole from below and two pulling up above, and my bottom bumping on every rock and stone.

Before midday we had covered twenty-four miles and reached

the Catholic Mission at Kitangali and I was thankful to stop and rest. As I hobbled slowly on my crutches to the door of the mission-house old Father Patrick (Dom Patrick Mühlbauer, O.S.B.) came out to meet me. He gave me one look and said "Cheer up! It's the way to Heaven." Then he took me in and made me wonderfully comfortable. He revived me with a bottle of home-made pineapple wine and gave me a meal. After that I slept for hours. Next morning at three o'clock we left the good Father and continued our jolting pilgrimage. We did another twenty-five miles that day, coming down the long hill off the plateau again into the Lukuledi valley, and at last reached Mtama where two years before the Indian driver had changed his radiator and regaled me with curry. Here was a small post-office (since abolished), and on its verandah I pitched my camp-bed and rested. There were rumours of a lorry somewhere in the vicinity, and the main road was said to be more or less passable as far as the head of the creek at Ming'oyo, so I waited. I camped on the post-office verandah all that day and night, but towards noon the next day the lorry arrived and I thankfully climbed on board, together with two missionary companions whom I had found at Mtama in a tent. We had a muddy and erratic ride, but eventually reached Ming'oyo and found a motor-boat going to Lindi. Four weeks later I was back in England and busy making plans for Lulindi hospital.

9

Building my First Hospital

In the dusk of a November evening in 1937 I was again in the train to Dover. I had found England good and suffered a momentary pang at leaving, but the cold of winter had begun, and anyway the job had now claimed me completely and I never for a moment dreamed of not renewing the contract. Had I known then that this was to be my last sight of England for eight years, my mood would doubtless have been more subdued.

Going on board the *Llandaff Castle* at Genoa, the first person I met was Lord Baden-Powell, the Chief Scout. Lady Baden-Powell spotted the Scout badge in my button-hole. There were many Scouts and Guides on board incognito and eventually we had a big party with the old Chief. At every port the local Scouts came out in launches, the Chief was taken ashore even before the ship was cleared, and was received by a guard of honour fit for a king. It was his last journey to Africa, and the last time I saw him.

The ship reached Tanga on Christmas Eve, so I broke my journey to spend Christmas day with my cousin Neil (now Bishop R. N. Russell, Superior of the Community of the Transfiguration), who was then pioneering a new mission at Mazinde, 100 miles inland. The train did not leave till the evening, so I went to wait at the town mission. After lunch they offered me a bed for siesta, and as it was unbearably hot I gladly accepted. I lay down and in a minute I was covered with small crawling things which I brushed off idly thinking they were just *dudus* (a *dudu* is any insect, or insignificant creature). They kept on coming, hundreds of them, and suddenly I realised that they were fleas. I spent the next two hours in the bath getting rid of them, during which time I caught something like two hundred on my clothes, my person, and the bathroom floor. They went down the drain as a brown sediment. Meanwhile two men were dealing with the bed, where doubtless hundreds more perished. Later I found that—unofficially—a cat had been bringing up its family on the bed. I thus lost my afternoon rest and acquired an extensive itch instead.

The train journey was a novel experience, as at that time we had no railway in the South. The ancient German coaches were alive with mosquitoes, so before the train started a man worked a powerful pyrethrum spray in the compartments, evicting not only the mosquitoes but for some time the passengers too. The track was rough (it has since been relaid) and the train rattled, banged and swayed violently as we progressed at about 20 m.p.h.

We stopped at every station—five minutes at the smaller ones and half an hour at the bigger ones. At one of the latter opportunity was taken to serve dinner, so that at least the soup would not be spilt. As it was Christmas Eve, the dinner included turkey and Christmas pudding with brandy sauce, quite good. The meal was not provided by the railway company, but by an Indian trader who had hired the dining car and made what he could out of it. We reached Mazinde at midnight, having taken six hours to cover 100 miles. The tiny station was lit by a single oil lamp, by the light of which a two-man band was playing. Someone said "They're drunk". Anyhow, they soon packed up and went away, and so did the train on its long crawl to Moshi. I fell in with some locals and walked the half mile or so to the Mission under a blaze of stars.

I arrived as midnight mass was ending, and spent a happy Christmas with Neil, who was living cheerfully in a very primitive hut in the village. He had come to Africa in 1933, working first in Salisbury, Rhodesia. He found the political and social situation there unbearable, and after a year transferred to Zanzibar. He had subsequently been working in Korogwe and Zigualand with his headquarters at Kideleko, before opening the new mission at Mazinde, from which he opened outstations further and further north extending to Mkomazi, Kihurio, and beyond. When the war caused the removal of German Lutheran missionaries in the Pare country, he took over much of their work as well. To do all this travelling he only had a bicycle; he never possessed a car, and would have been embarrassed by anything so grand.

On first leaving for Africa he had suddenly remembered the poverty of St. Francis Xavier, and had given away the boxes he had so carefully prepared and packed. Instead he had left Edinburgh with a large holdall and the clothes he stood up in, the station platform packed with a crowd which began singing hymns but broke down into tears. His persistent simplicity of living and frugality was an example to us all, even when he was transferred to the town parish of Tanga, and was eventually made a bishop with charge of the islands of Zanzibar and Pemba.

There was plenty of life at Mazinde, including mosquitoes. Neil's little church stands to this day, but his hut has long ago fallen down. After a pleasant couple of days in his company I made my way back to Tanga and from there to the south by sea.

I reached Lulindi with plans for a proper hospital, and some money to start building it. The biggest share came from a legacy of the late Dr. Culver James, sometimes President of the Guild of St. Luke, and the hospital was to be his memorial. During the rains it was impossible to make a start, but as soon as they were ended I got busy making bricks again. At that time we used only 'green' or sun-dried bricks, under the mistaken impression that burning bricks was costly and difficult. This was a pity. The green bricks were marvellously hard, as long as they remained dry, and could resist driving rain, but they could not stand up to being quietly soaked by a steady trickle of water, and consequently a leaking roof could demolish a building in a short time. Our grass roofs were therefore a constant anxiety, and during the rains I was always running round looking for dangerous leaks and underpinning beams where a wall or pillar showed signs of giving way. Eventually I tried burning some bricks, and when I found how cheap and easy it was I wished we had done it from the beginning. But by that time the greater part of the hospital was built.

The first building to go up, after the operating theatre, was the main outpatient building, including the dispensary and laboratory. This building I set squarely on a vacant patch in the middle of the hospital area, and the rest of the hospital subsequently aligned itself upon it. The plan was cruciform, with maximum roof-span to the limbs in order to introduce as much light and air as possible. This was enhanced by having no ceilings, and a big open verandah in front, which served as a waiting room. The open roof attracted bats, owls and swallows, and we had to put up a large quantity of wire-netting to deter them. An important feature of the new building was a built-in stove, on which instruments could be sterilised, and water boiled and distilled. The stove was fired from outside, burning uncut logs which were fed in gradually and gave off a great heat.

When I had been marking out the foundations for this building—one evening in May, after ordinary working hours—my assistant was a young patient, a schoolboy with a malignant tumour of the jaw, for which he was awaiting operation the next morning. He was cheerful and unconcerned, and quite absorbed in what we were doing. It was as well that he did not know how nervous I felt, since it was the first time I had undertaken the removal of a whole upper jaw. He made an uneventful recovery and went home as cheerful as ever, and later, with the help of the District Commissioner, I was able to send him to Dar es Salaam, where the Government dental surgeon fitted him out with a fine set of new teeth. When he returned he was an object of great interest in the village. Not only had he gone all the way to Dar es

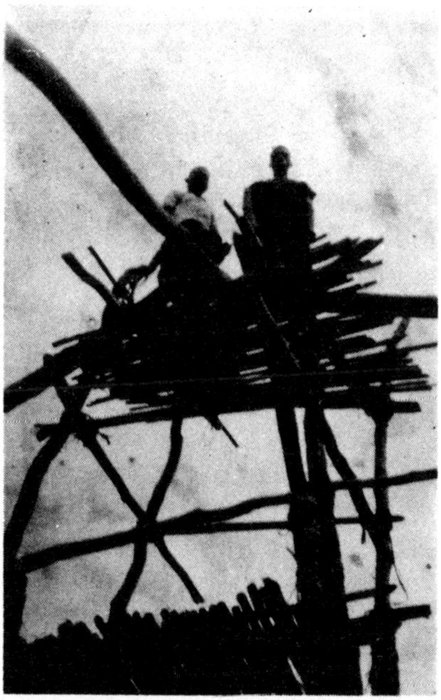

Building Lulindi Hospital: *above*, erecting the central roof truss; *below*, brick-making—filling the moulds.

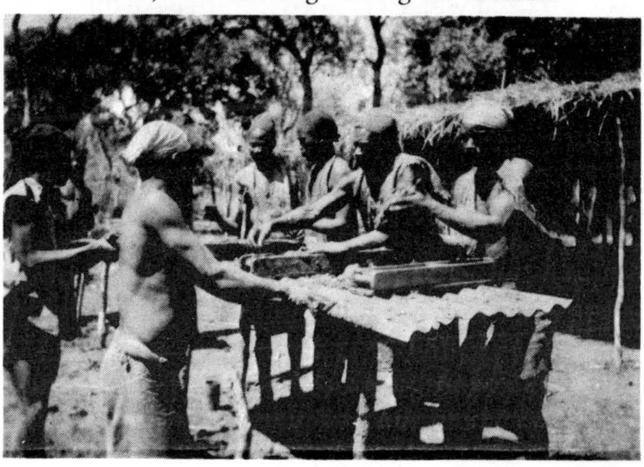

Salaam and returned alive, but he had teeth which would come out and go in again. Also he had a new shirt.

The building he had helped to measure was the largest and most ambitious brick structure in Lulindi. Before the end of the year we had moved in, and felt great satisfaction as we worked in such unaccustomed space. Patients continued to flock in as usual, many making no secret of having come only to see the new hospital. We still had no proper wards for the patients, but I was not anxious to build these too soon until we had more trained nurses and an improvement in local standards of hygiene. It was better to keep the sick and their relatives in the huts, where at least a dirty family would only dirty their own hut and not a whole ward. (I added wards some years later, when we had an adequate nursing staff.) Meanwhile, however, I had other work on hand.

There was nothing now to prevent us from building the much needed hospital at Newala, so I started on this at the same time as the Lulindi one, commuting between them as best I could. I concentrated on Lulindi, as the Sister in charge at Newala was supremely capable (if only, said her Superior, Sister Anne had been a man!) and with her senior dresser Petro Manyamba as overseer, had the outpatient building and patients' huts rising quickly. To decrease the water-problem in future, I roofed the Newala hospital with corrugated iron, so that we could collect rain-water in tanks, and the extra expense was well worthwhile.

The major problem in starting to build at Newala was the lack of water, as has already been explained, and the earth of the plateau was quite useless for making bricks. In the end I had the bricks made in the valley, where there was not only water but good clay, and then contracted with two local chiefs to have them carried up. In this way I evaded what would have been an impossible operation with casual labour. The chiefs were wary at first, but when we had fixed a reasonable lump sum for the job they became less reluctant, and the 35,000 bricks came up the 1,000 feet on the heads of their people. They were pleased to receive so large a sum in hard cash, but their enjoyment had probably lost its edge by the time they had finished the colossal wrangle which took place when they attempted to share out the money according to the number of bricks each man had carried. I was glad to be out of it!

We allowed for an eventual total of fifty beds, every one of which was usually filled, but the bulk of the work remained with outpatients, owing to the thick population and the readiness of the Wamakonde to walk long distances. We were soon having 300 attendances on busy days, which grew over the years to 400 and even 500 and more.

The technique for dealing with these crowds was as follows. When the hospital was complete we had a staff of two sisters, two African Medical Assistants, one African nurse, and about four dressers. One Sister and one Medical Assistant examined and prescribed for the patients, the second medical assistant made microscopic diagnoses, and the rest of the staff carried out the treatments. Work began at 8 a.m., when there was already a crowd waiting. At about 1 p.m. half the staff went to get some food and the rest carried on. The great aim was to dispose of the morning patients before 3 p.m., when the afternoon session began, but often it became a continous performance. At three o'clock the staff who had fed and rested returned to work and the others went to eat. All being well the last patients were usually disposed of by 6 p.m. The same staff had meanwhile to be dealing with the fifty in-patients as well. Even when the doctor was there things were no easier, as there would be special consultations to make and operations to do.

At Lulindi we had at last got our first fully trained Medical Assistant, the late Imanuel Chitenje, who was able to take a large and increasing share of responsibility. Being an entirely new species of worker at that time, he did not find his life easy at first, but he soon proved his worth, and not only in his technical work. Late one night a small girl was brought in with a rare and very fatal type of meningitis (due to the so-called Influenza Bacillus). She was comatose and the outlook seemed hopeless, but we were then experimenting with our very limited stocks of Prontosil, and I thought there was a chance that the new drug might save the child's life. At Lulindi our small supply of injectable Prontosil was already finished, but there was a very small amount at Masasi. To send a porter for it would take fourteen hours or more, and the child would certainly be dead by the time he returned. But Imanuel was a great cyclist, who had actually bent the cranks of his bicycle by his furious riding, and he was willing to go for it. He left at 1 a.m. in pitch darkness for a journey of fifty-eight miles along footpaths and tracks that in England would be thought bad even for walking. The rains had just finished, and had left the roads in an appalling state with lumps of bare rock, drifts of sand, swamps, deep holes and unbridged streams and rivers. There was also the chance of meeting a leopard on the way. At Masasi he stopped only long enough to collect the precious drug and was off again. At 10.30 a.m. he came riding furiously into the hospital, streaming with sweat and covered with burrs from the tangled bush. The child was still alive then, but even Prontosil could not perform the miracle required, and Imanuel's great ride had been in vain.

Meningitis, of several varieties, was a recurring problem and often fatal. On a journey to the west, beyond Tunduru, I found a schoolboy being nursed in a dispensary. He had acute meningitis, and was already in coma. Lumbar-puncture and the microscope revealed the pneumococcus: a very poor outlook. The only anti-pneumococcal drug available was sulphapyridine (the famous M.&B. 693) in tablet form. However, although apparently comatose he still had a swallowing reflex, so we crushed the tablets in milk and a devoted Sister sat by him day and night feeding him the mixture with a teaspoon. I started on the usual four-hourly routine with 1½ grammes each time, but he got rapidly worse. I stepped up the dosage until he was having 2 grammes every two hours—drastic, but it was kill or cure and he survived it. His temperature gradually fell, and the dreaded convulsions did not appear, but after two weeks he was still unconscious, and the good Sister was almost worn out. Then the Bishop came to see him, and while he was there, the boy suddenly opened his eyes. After that he returned rapidly to normal, but there was a startling consequence. Having previously been a very troublesome boy with a bad reputation at school and at home, he was now docile, pleasant and with charming manners, a complete personality change. Nor was his intellect impaired. He subsequently obtained a responsible job which he holds to this day. He had undergone, unintentionally but very successfully, the treatment of prolonged deep unconsciousness, which was then being advocated for difficult mental cases.

Besides building up the two main hospitals I was opening up more dispensaries in strategic places. With medical aid so scarce these dispensaries filled a great need, dealing with much of the minor ailments, not infrequently saving life, and acting as collecting centres for serious cases needing transfer to hospital. One of these new dispensaries was at Mkunya, on the Makonde plateau, so placed that it was able to take over work from overpressed Newala and Mahuta, and also save sick people many weary miles travelling. In the rains I used to visit Mkunya by bicycle, a journey of eight miles, downhill all the way, a lovely run—but uphill all the way back.

The second new dispensary was at Chihako, a remote spot on the Ruvuma river and twenty miles beyond our small hospital at Luatala. The road was the roughest of bush tracks, passable with caution in a car at 10 m.p.h. in dry weather. In the rains it was a walk through an intimidating length of overgrown forest where civilisation seemed very far away, especially after the sun had gone down. On my second visit I walked down to see the great Ruvuma. The way lay along the dry bed of a tributary, which was dotted all over with footprints of lion, hippo, elephant and all kinds of smaller animals. The Ruvuma itself was a magnificent sight. I had often seen it from the hilltops, far off, but even so I was amazed at its size and beauty. It was half a mile from bank to bank, the water clear and blue, flowing swiftly in three channels between banks of silver sand. Tumbled rocky hills and forest came right down to the water's edge, and in mid-stream there was an occasional wooded island. In the dry weather the river could be forded in places, with care, though a canoe was a safer means of crossing, but in the rains it filled up from bank to bank and sometimes overflowed, covering the land with a wilderness of water that deposited hippos in fields and swept away villages with their inhabitants. One poor woman was carried downstream about thirty miles on the floating roof of her house, until at last it went ashore and she was rescued.

The dispensary itself was the simplest imaginable—a one-roomed hut with a small verandah, built by the people of the village. It had only just been opened when it was narrowly missed by a whirlwind which came suddenly out of the forest and wrecked the village school close by. The roof of the school went straight up in the air and came down all over the play-ground. The whirlwind went twisting away with all the dogs barking at it, and disappeared in someone's plantation.

10
Chihako and Elsewhere

The following fragment of diary for 1938 may shed a little light on my daily activities at that time.

Monday, October 24th Left Newala for Lulindi. Arrived at 8.30 a.m. and found everything at a standstill owing to a wedding just coming out of church with much firing of guns, singing and dancing. Dealt with a crowd of patients in hospital, including a good many of the wedding guests who had dropped in, until at 10.45 a.m. the Bishop of Nyasaland arrived from Masasi with Dr. Taylor. Drove the Bishop to Luatala for lunch, saw a few patients and returned to Lulindi for tea. Bishop impressed with new hospital buildings, especially roof. Changed cars with Dr. Taylor, as hers looked incapable of reaching Nyasaland intact. Departure of Bishop and Dr. Taylor for Masasi and Lake Nyasa.

Tuesday, October 25th Operation day: two operations booked; one patient's father consented but didn't turn up; the other patient's father turned up but would not consent, so both operations postponed. Spent a busy morning in hospital and on buildings. Afternoon left in Dr. Taylor's car for monthly visit to Chihako. Stopped at Luatala for tea and to pick up medicine chest. Car making curious noises. . . . Proceeded sedately and arrived safely at Chihako about sunset.

Wednesday, October 26th Good crowd of patients at dispensary at 8 a.m., but early prospects not maintained, grand total thirty only; some had walked six hours to get there. Although numbers are still small there are signs that this new station should prove worthwhile when there is a resident dresser. Afternoon: attempted repair of car.

Thursday, October 27th Patients not so early or so many. Some had arrived overnight from many miles away in Mozambique, but had never seen a white man, and when the time came their courage failed them, and they went home again unseen and untreated!

Booked a neighbouring chief for operation at Lulindi—he *may* arrive—and caused a sensation by producing a photograph of the local chief and family taken on a previous visit. Got away at 10.15 a.m., leaving a dresser to follow up for a few days, and steered for Mikindani, 130 miles away. Car behaved well for a mile, but the rough road [just a pair of ruts through the forest] soon loosened up all the trouble again, and by Luatala we were rattling and grinding horribly. Decided further repairs would take too long, so pushed on cautiously and reached Newala [1,500 feet higher] for lunch, without mishap. After lunch continued on a "good" road for 30 miles to Tandahimba, where a rear tyre burst with astonishing violence: 12-inch rent in a new inner tube and the hub-disc went flying off into a field. The noise brought out one of our nurses who was waiting to be collected. Told her the car was likely to break up and must spend an hour or so on repairs if we were to reach Mikindani at all. At this point an Indian lorry appeared, going to Mikindani and looking quite new, so packed nurse on to it and turned back to Newala. Car now became rapidly worse. . . . Crawled on another mile at 5 m.p.h. and turned into Mission at Nanhyanga. Found Father Emilius in occupation and a very convenient pit in front of the house, excavated at some time for building material, i.e. mud. Ran car over pit and went to bed.

Friday, October 28th. As church was being entirely rebuilt . . . Father Emilius said Mass in front room of teacher's house. Delightful and homely sight of teacher's youngest child, stark naked, crawling happily across the floor from Mother, in the congregation, to Father serving at the altar. This is a strongly Muslim district, with no Christians as yet but the two teachers and their families, so these with Simon and myself formed the congregation. After breakfast stripped to the waist and got in the pit. Wrestled with universal joint for 3½ hours, but finally victorious. Intense interest throughout on part of small crowd of children, to detriment of school attendance. By 11.30 was nearly as black as they were, had a stand-up bath and returned to Newala, car running fairly well.

Saturday, October 29th. Inspected new hospital buildings and had serious argument with carpenter over disposition of beams. Adjourned the matter and was busily dealing with patients when a messenger arrived from Luatala; had been walking since 1 a.m. and lost the way. Message reported a "crocodile case" needing urgent attention, so left remaining patients to Sister and set off for Luatala. Found the patient was a child, who while stooping down to wash in the river had been slashed in the face by a crocodile's tail which had torn his nose half off down to the bone, ripped up his cheek into the mouth and crushed his lower jaw into three pieces. The general effect was that all one side of his face had slipped, besides being frightfully lacerated. The Sister gave a very skilful anaesthetic and I repaired the damage as well as I could. Then after seeing a few more patients I returned to Newala.

Sunday, October 30th. While taking a stroll round the new hospital buildings after Mass found two strangers looking lost. One was quite blind and the other had led him all the way from Mikindani, ninety miles, on foot, to get medicine. It was the more pathetic as his blindness was probably due to a cerebral tumour and there was nothing to do for him.

Monday, October 31st. Settled dispute with carpenter and spent some time selecting and measuring beams for the roof. Dealt with the usual Monday crowd of patients till about 1 p.m. A few more after tea, and then off by car to see a reported case of possible pneumonia a couple of miles away. Whole village gathered on doorstep in respectful silence to watch the magic ceremonial of the stethoscope. Decided patient had only got fibrositis after all, so left him some medicine and came away.

Tuesday, November 1st. All Saints' Day, normally kept as a holiday like a Sunday, but Tuesday happens to be the day for the weekly dispensary at Mkunya and it was not practicable to close this, so all to Mass first and then off as quickly as possible in the car—one Sister, two dressers, one clerk, Simon and myself. Before we left, another crocodile case had arrived, a man with the front of his knee bitten right off. Gave instructions to remaining Sister and then off to Mkunya arriving about 10 a.m. Most of the patients had gone away, but hearing the car they soon came back and we worked till 2 p.m., dealing with about a hundred. One girl with a bad ulcer following smallpox needed in-patient treatment, so after lunch we loaded her into the car and brought her back to Newala. The thrill of a car-ride is often a sufficient lure to get into hospital patients who would otherwise not come. When just about to start I found the patient's brother was proposing to come too. As he was still infectious from smallpox I turned him out. . . . [Smallpox has at last been completely eradicated from Tanzania.]

Wednesday, November 2nd. Off at 6.30 a.m. for Mahuta, where we also have a dispensary, but with two resident dressers. Took a Sister and another dresser for the day. Quite a busy morning; 120 patients altogether. The recognised offering for a course of injections is 50 cents [sixpence]. Was somewhat troubled by one group of patients who had each brought 50 cents but had no need of injections, and others who needed injections but had not brought 50 cents! The senior dresser there is an excellent missionary and has done great work at Mahuta, a difficult place with a strong Moslem population, rather hostile. Now as a reward I am sending him to Chihako as the beginning of a resident medical staff there. It is a place of great possibilities, but it is very remote from his own people and it will not be easy. Before returning to Newala we loaded up a large sack of corn [offerings in kind], an empty 40-gallon drum, and a bundle of live hens [also offerings]. The car being small we put the hens in the drum, where they rode safely though without much of a view.

Thursday, November 3rd. More building and then a steady stream of patients, finishing by pulling out several teeth with anaesthesia. Afternoon: weekly mail sent off, then twice-weekly lecture to dressers and then to the Boma to get some news from the District Officer's wireless set, the only one between Lindi and Tunduru.

Friday, November 4th. Building again; then loaded the car with 400 lbs. of Portland cement, eleven sheets of corrugated iron, and a crate of glass, and prepared to leave Newala. Having heard that a Government M.O. had arrived at the rest camp seeking solitude and Newala air as a cure for lumbago and sciatica, I went to call and express sympathy. M.O. asked for advice; I suggested manipulation under anaesthesia. Suggestion promptly accepted and carried out. M.O. no featherweight: quite exhausting. Left at 2 p.m. and returned to Lulindi. Dealt with urgent cases and inspected new buildings.

Saturday, November 5th. Morning on buildings, measuring new boundary fence, visiting stone quarry and seeing patients in the intervals. Afternoon: about to set out to visit a smallpox case when a lorry arrived with a policeman and a corpse from 50 miles away. Post-mortem wanted at once. Did post-mortem and sent dispenser to see smallpox case. Wrote report and body removed by lorry for burial. Junior nurse retired to bed with malaria. 4.30 p.m. delayed start for Luatala, carrying eleven sheets of corrugated iron in car for roofing new store. Deposited same and saw several cases, notably the crocodile child. A nasty mess, but condition very good all things considered. Returned Lulindi 7.30 p.m., car lights working intermittently. Microscope work and accounts until bedtime.

Sunday, November 6th. A very moving incident at Mass. After the sermon a Christian who had fallen away to Islam returned and asked for penance that he might be restored to the Church. He repeated his baptismal vows, made years ago, he re-affirmed the Creed, and then he made public confession ". . . that I denied the Lord Christ and followed Muhammad". These lapses of Christians to Islam are very hard to change, so the return of this man today is a matter for real thanksgiving.

That was two consecutive weeks, and quite enough. So much travelling is very detrimental to systematic work in hospital. What couldn't one have done with another doctor!

I had great hopes for Chihako, but after a couple of years the people all moved back across the river whence they had come, and it was quickly swallowed up again by the forest.

Until 1939 I had been dependent on casual motor transport when motoring was possible at all, the old ambulance having finally been pensioned off due to old age and rust. Now, however, my sister in England rallied support from many good friends, and raised the money to buy a serviceable ambulance. In great excitement I went to Lindi to see it being landed from the ship and drove it away in triumph. It was a powerful six-cylinder Chevrolet, very strongly built with a long plywood body and tail-door. The sides were open, with canvas curtains against sun and rain. I had lockers built on, and for nine years it carried me, my patients, my staff, our supplies, even livestock on occasion, through mud and water, sand and bush, all over southern Tanzania. It never let me down, although I always carried a rope, a spade, an axe, chains for the wheels, and the huge instrument known as a "Tanganyika jack". With this emergency equipment on board we went anywhere, even places where there was no road at all, and the service of these remote dispensaries in particular was made much easier.

11
Scouting in the Bush

Until I came to Africa, much of my spare time had been taken up with Scouting. I had been a Scout since the age of eleven, and was expecting to continue in Africa where I had left off in England. However, I was disappointed to find that there were no Scouts in the whole of Southern Tanganyika. More accurately, there was one, George Tibbatts, a young missionary who had arrived armed with a Commissioner's warrant and the intention of starting Scouting in a big way. However, he had met so much active discouragement from those who thought they knew better, and notably from his bishop, that he had been unable even to make a beginning. The Bishop, who had left England when the Scout movement had been in existence only a year, was sure it would be a disturbing influence and quite unsuitable for African boys. Those of the older missionaries who knew anything about Scouting dismissed it impatiently on the grounds that African boys "knew it already". I was personally not impressed by these opinions, but as I was new to the country I decided to bide my time until I was at least fluent in the local language and knew something of customs and local background. Meanwhile I gave all the moral support I could to the Commissioner, and whenever we met we discussed how and when we could make a start.

Eventually, after nearly five years, George succeeded in wearing down the Bishop's opposition and received permission to start in a small way. He began with a group of boys from the school (Chidya) of which he was headmaster, and enrolled the first of them on Coronation Day, 1937. Unfortunately, he broke his leg six months later while on leave and never returned to Africa. I succeeded him as Commissioner, but living twenty miles from the school I could not take over his troop. No one else was forthcoming, and in the end I had the melancholy duty of closing it down.

Meanwhile, however, I was laying plans for a new start at Lulindi. This needed much thought and preparation, because not only were the older missionaries opposed to the idea, but none of the African population had the slightest idea what Boy Scouts were. Worse than that, the word Scout, spelt "*Skauti*", was known from the First World War as meaning a military spy. I found, however, that Imanuel the dispenser had once seen some Scouts in Zanzibar. He had also read about B.P. So with his help I collected half a dozen young men whom I already knew well, and early in 1939 formed a small Rover crew. I had to explain everything from the very beginning, but they lapped it up, and on Palm Sunday I was able to invest them as Rovers. I did it with a soaring temperature, and as soon as the ceremony was over I retired to bed, but the seed had been sown.

From the first I made it clear to my young Rovers that their job of Rover service was to be to introduce Scouting to the boys of Lulindi. In fact they introduced it to the whole Southern Province of Tanganyika. In August that year, more than 100 boys were camped in the forest undergoing an initiation rite. This seemed to be just the right moment, so the Rovers visited the camp and put on an attractive display of Scout games and skills. I finished with a short talk, and invited any boys who were interested to come along to a meeting, as soon as they were out of the initiation camp, and see for themselves. A large number of boys put their names down, and we fixed the date for 4 September. Hitler got in first, and on 3 September war was declared. The parents said "What did we tell you? It's all a trick to get our boys away to the war!" Scouting at Lulindi was nearly killed at birth that day, but five small boys, mostly of the naughtier type, were sufficiently independent to turn up and see for themselves. The Rovers remained solidly loyal and so the troop got going. After a week or two the adventurous five managed to persuade some of their young friends to risk parental disapproval and join, and eventually we are able to form two complete patrols.

Our Scouting in the beginning was very simple, naturally with a strong African flavour, and so it has remained. We always met out of doors, as B.P. originally intended, and our headquarters was a small place in the forest which we cleared for ourselves. There each patrol built itself a hut of bamboo and grass, there we hoisted our flag (of St. George, the Union Jack being a foreign emblem) on an ebony pole that we had cut and carted from the forest, and there we met; but having met we often ranged far and wide through the forest, along the stream, round the villages, coming back to our clearing before sunset for a bath in the stream. If we wanted a short camp we simply camped there, sleeping in the huts or even under the stars.

We had a simplified uniform made locally to keep down expense, but I insisted that the Scouts must pay for it. They looked very smart and soon became an object of intense interest to those boys who were still afraid to join. We made our own staves, flags, belts and whistles, buying only the official badges. When it came to choosing patrol names there was some difficulty. The Scouts were rather chary of the usual Lions or Panthers, as such savage beasts had a bad name locally. They all wanted to be Rabbits on account of the "Brer Rabbit" tradition in African folklore, but I could not agree to that as Brer Rabbit is always a twister. In the end they plumped for Sheep and Pigs.

After some weeks the Sheep got rather tired of their farmyard appellation, especially when the Pigs shouted "worms!" at them, and quietly changed it for something more ferocious, but the Pigs survived for years and eventually covered themselves with glory by defeating all comers from thirty troops at a district rally.

In spite of my faith in Scouting, I had introduced it at Lulindi with at least some degree of anxiety as to how acceptable it would be, and how much modification there would have to be. I need not have worried. The reactions of my African Scouts were almost invariably the same as those of my London Scouts. They liked the same games, disliked the same things, and danced to B.P.'s piping as readily as boys anywhere. One of the pleasantest developments was that two of the more senior missionaries, Archdeacon Donald Parsons and Canon Harry Denniss, who had been almost hostile to the introduction of Scouting and openly sceptical of its value, eventually became our most devoted supporters and went to great lengths to promote and facilitate Scouting for the boys in their respective parishes.

The first year of Scouting had its ups and downs, with parental opposition still to be reckoned with. However, the year passed, and we felt strong enough to make our first expedition outside the parish. We headed for the Ruvuma river, some twenty miles away, and had a never-to-be-forgotten day camping on the bank under a great shady tree, swimming, canoeing, fishing and eating food that we had cooked ourselves. Late in the evening we headed for home and stopped half-way for the night at Luatala. We were kindly entertained and on the next day, which was a Sunday, were in church in uniform. Afterwards there was something approaching a riot, the parish priest (Canon Parsons, mentioned above) being besieged by a crowd of boys demanding "who are these beautiful strangers?" and "why can't we have this game here?" The upshot was that a vigorous troop came into being at Luatala, where there seemed to be fewer inhibitions than at Lulindi. The only trouble was that I had to run it, as well as the Lulindi troop, myself. I did this by having a meeting every Thursday afternoon after my weekly visit to the Luatala dispensary. I usually spent the night and returned to Lulindi early on Friday morning.

News of the Luatala troop spread rapidly, and there were demands for troops from all over the place. I could not run any more myself, so after Christmas I arranged a small training course, quite unofficial, at which I put across the elements of Scoutmastership to a dozen likely young men. With these I was able to start up several more troops, and at Easter a second training course allowed further expansion. By this time several of the missionaries, with previous experience of Scouting in England, began to come forward and join in, including Robin Lamburn, then Warden of the diocesan theological college, one of the most brilliant leaders of Scouts I have ever met. The movement thus spread much further afield.

By the middle of 1941 we had about a dozen troops in action, and I decided it was time to have a district rally. This was a great success, and since then has been a highly popular annual event, providing a meeting-point and stimulus for isolated troops who never otherwise see another Scout all the year round. That first rally at Lulindi was modest enough, lasting only twenty-four hours (later they sometimes ran to five days) with less than two hundred Scouts, but it made a lasting impression on the local people and was an eye-opener to many of the missionaries. The Mother Superior was heard to say that she would never have believed she would live to see two hundred African boys all doing the same thing at the same time, and in such good order!

As for the Bishop, we made him guest-of-honour and had him in the centre of everything, quite literally when we put him at the middle of a wheel-rally and two hundred Scouts burst from the bushes and rushed at him from all sides, yelling and brandishing their staves. They stopped dead a measured two yards from him and gave him a chief's salute. His anxious expression gave place to a smile of relief and a gracious reply. Scouting had come to stay.

12
Further and Further Afield

Although my most distant regular dispensary was only forty-five miles away, I sometimes travelled further afield and gave casual medical help at remote places where there was no hospital or dispensary within reach. In particular I sometimes used to take the Archdeacon, Donald Parsons, in the ambulance (he never had a car) to tour the further parts of his archdeaconry, and while he was visiting schools I would deal with patients by the roadside, dosing malaria, extracting teeth, and suchlike. One day while so employed in a small village more than 100 miles from home, I noticed a number of men gathered on the Headman's doorstep. A messenger said "When you have finished, there is a matter awaiting you." I went over, and was told that they had decided I must open a dispensary there forthwith. I said that nothing would please me more, only I had neither the time nor the money. I suggested they should approach the District Commissioner.

Rather to my surprise they did so. The District Commissioner replied that he had no medical staff available, but would be prepared to help the mission doctor with funds if he would find the staff. In the end a unique arrangement was concluded whereby the local authority should provide a suitable building and pay all expenses (supplies, salaries, upkeep, etc.) with myself finding the staff, ordering the drugs and giving general supervision. This seemed to suit everyone. The building was a disused court-house, very solidly built, at a place called Mchicha (meaning spinach), a good centre of population and remote from any other medical help. I transferred two dressers from other dispensaries, ordered all the necessary equipment and drugs, and had the place suitably redecorated. The District Commissioner had agreed that I should have a free hand in the running of the unit, on the same lines as a mission dispensary, but when all was ready for the opening he suddenly said that of course the staff must not pray before starting work. (Such prayers were in no way compulsory for the patients, most of whom were non-Christians.) I replied that in view of the agreement I could not accept any such restrictions. He was adamant, so I said politely that I was sorry it would not be possible to open the dispensary as planned. He was very upset, and said "Then I think you had better see the Provincial Commissioner." "I will" I said, and left him. He then proceeded to telephone the P.C., but the line was out of order, so when I reached the P.C.'s office next day he had heard nothing. I told him my story and he said "The man's a fool. I'll write to him." The dispensary was opened as planned, and the District Commissioner thereafter proved most co-operative. It was such a success that next year the local authority asked me to undertake another on the same terms. This was specially built, at Kitaya, a very remote spot on the banks of the Ruvuma, where the hippos grunted in the evening and the elephants trumpeted at dawn.

Visiting these remote dispensaries was time-consuming, and the long bumpy sandy road over the Makonde plateau was a weary trail, but the outstanding success of both dispensaries made it well worthwhile. At least the long journey was rarely without incident, even if only a boiling radiator on a waterless stretch, or a total failure of the lights after dark. One day a pack of wild dogs danced in front of the car, big multi-coloured spotted creatures with the sunlight shining through their large pink ears. Another time, after dark on a lonely stretch, I met a small group of men carrying a rough hammock. I stopped to investigate. There was a woman lying in the hammock, in a bad way, and when I lifted her covering I saw a heap of bowels underneath. "Her husband ripped her up" they said "and escaped across the river. We are taking her to the hospital at Mikindani." As the journey was some forty miles, the chances of her arriving alive were poor. The party gladly accepted a lift in the ambulance, so we loaded her in and I turned round and made for the Benedictine Mission at Nanyamba, only about twenty-five miles away. It was not one of my dispensaries, but it was the nearest place with any facilities for operating and the case was desperate. We were there by about 9 p.m. and called out the somewhat startled Father Superior (the late Dom Ursus Forster, O.S.B.). He made us welcome, and brought his Aladdin lamp to the dispensary while the dispenser prepared his meagre equipment. There was a massive table on which he dispensed his medicines, so we cleared off the bottles and put the patient on one end of it and a bowl of lysol on the other. There were no sterile towels or dressings, so we boiled pieces of old linen and soaked swabs in lysol. I had a few instruments with me and a bottle of chloroform. I handed this to the dispenser, and while he kept the patient efficiently anaesthetised I managed to remove the worst of the dirt from the bowels and put them back where they belonged. Mercifully there was no perforation. I sewed her up with ordinary thread, and left her for the dispenser to nurse. She developed pneumonia, which he successfully treated, but the wound gave no trouble and she went home in good form.

This belly-ripping was not uncommon and usually, though not always, it was the act of an outraged husband who suspected his wife's fidelity. One such husband, however, simply took a machete and hacked his wife all over. He then ran away, and she was brought in to Lulindi hospital a lacerated mess. Some of the cuts had gone right into the bone of her skull, and one had severed her upper lip from side to side. Altogether I sewed up twenty-seven cuts, but the patient never turned a hair. She was much more hurt in spirit than in body, and wept with mortification at having been caught by her husband with another man. However, her wounds healed uneventfully, and by the time she left for home she had quite regained her composure. How she had escaped death, after twenty-seven blows with a sharp and heavy machete was a mystery. I can only suppose that the husband was so angry that he did not stop to take proper aim.

Nocturnal emergencies were fortunately not very frequent at Lulindi, but when they came they did not lack variety. One evening I was drinking coffee after dinner when a face looked in at the window and said "You'd better come out here. We've got a man with his brains running out". I took this light-heartedly as dramatic hyperbole, but when outside I was shocked to see that it was the literal truth. They had put down a portable bed just outside the window, and on it lay a young man, apparently unconscious. His scalp was split and torn, and from the wounds brain matter dripped slowly to the ground.

There was one of the all-too-frequent food shortages just then (famine, in plain English) and apparently a cane-rat had been spotted in a tree. Food! Someone had cut down the tree to get the animal, and the tree had fallen squarely on this young man's head, smashing it like an egg. When I had him on the operating table I saw his skull was in five pieces, and as I tried to manoeuvre them into place more brain kept oozing out. However, at last the jig-saw was complete and the scalp sewn up. To everyone's surprise he made a quick recovery, and walked home. He seemed to have a rather simple and euphoric mentality, but his family said he had always been like that!

While he was lying in hospital he asked for, and received, Baptism. Serious illness has brought many people to make this great decision, which they might otherwise have put off for years or even for ever. Much has been said for and against Baptism of the sick ("taking the opportunity" or "taking advantage" of their sickness, according to one's viewpoint) and I shall not add to the controversy. Here, however, are two true stories of clinical Baptism, and you can draw what moral you like from them.

The first concerns the Yao chief Matola II. His predecessor: Matola I (not his father, but his maternal uncle, as Yao inheritance is matriarchal) was famous for having alone withstood the Angoni invasion of southern Tanganyika in the late nineteenth century, and having from the first welcomed and protected the Universities' Mission. Matola II, who was respected by both the German and the British governments for his strong rule, continued this policy, and eventually nearly all his people were Christians. He himself, however, had hung back until well on in life, when he became seriously ill and seemed to be dying. He was urged to receive Baptism before it was too late. "No" he said, "that would be cheating. I have held back all these years, and if I accept now for fear of dying, it will be like offering God a bribe. No, you can all pray for me, and if I die I will hope for the mercy of God. But if I get better, *then* I will be baptised to show my gratitude."

He did recover and was baptised, remaining a faithful and devout Christian to the end of his long life.

The second story concerns the late Father Norbert Wüst, one of the Benedictine pioneers in southern Tanganyika. At one time he opened a new mission at Mtua, in a strongly Muslim neighbourhood, and after some time became friendly with an old Muslim teacher living nearby. He had many discussions with this man, but he remained adamant in his faith. One day, as Father Norbert was leaving the old teacher's house, another priest who had accompanied him slipped him a holy medal of St. Benedict. "Try this" he said. Father Norbert took it, and as they passed through the door of the house he quietly inserted it over the lintel. He was observed, however, and later the old teacher discovered the medal. In great anger he carried it off to the nearest British government officer, who took a serious view. Father Norbert was soon summoned before the court of the Provincial Commissioner at Lindi, and charged with interfering in the Muslim teacher's religion. He pleaded "guilty" and was fined a substantial sum. This he flatly refused to pay. "Then you will have to go to prison" said the Provincial Commissioner, much affronted. "All right" said Father Norbert, "I'll go!" However, before he could be transported to the only prison which then accepted Europeans, some 400 miles away, the Bishop had intervened and paid his fine. Father Norbert was upset at being denied the chance of imprisonment for the Faith. Some time later the old teacher became seriously ill and sent for Father Norbert. "Father", he said, "you are my friend. I am dying, and I want to be baptised before I die. But my people must not know." So Father Norbert baptised him secretly, and he died a Christian.

Reverting to nocturnal emergencies: Mariam, a young teacher's wife, came in to Lulindi hospital to have her second baby. The birth of the first one had been so difficult that it seemed impossible for her to give birth to another without surgical assistance, probably caesarian section. However, she seemed to have some time to go, so I went on a planned routine visit to Newala. The road was closed by the rains, so I walked as usual. I had only been there one day when I was awakened at 3 a.m. by someone calling. It was a messenger from Lulindi to say Mariam was in labour. My heart sank. The messenger must have been on the road five hours already, and I had the same journey to do in the reverse direction, on foot. Ten hours of obstructed labour—anything might happen! I flung on some clothes, picked up a hurricane lamp, and ran, literally. I never saw the messenger again, but I hope he had some rest. I ran, I walked, I ran again. It was pitch dark, but I had my lamp; the road for the first seven miles was level and sandy, and I made good progress. Then I turned off along a narrow path through dense bush for another four miles, until I reached the top of the rocky staircase up which I had been dragged so painfully many years before.

This time I had two sound legs and down I went, slipping and slithering and jumping from rock to rock. At last I was down the thousand-foot escarpment and through the familiar woods at the foot. By this time day had broken and I put out my lamp. The last few miles were through cultivated fields and I ran on, beginning to sweat now with the rising sun. Almost at the mission I passed an old lady hoeing her field. She looked up. "What news Mama?" "It's a boy!" she called, and laughed all over her face. I could hardly believe it, so I pushed on to the hospital. It was quite true; a healthy boy and Mariam hadn't turned a hair. That she had delivered a full-size child *per vias naturales* was something approaching a miracle. With a strong sense of anti-climax I went and ate a large breakfast.

13
A Pioneer in Leprosy

I cannot take this story further without mentioning Edith Shelley, one of the most remarkable women who ever tramped the dusty roads of Tanganyika.

Edith Shelley, the daughter of a Lincolnshire vicar, with a classical education, joined the Universities' Mission as a trained nurse in 1923. She was very small, desperately short-sighted, but tough and independent to a sometimes embarrassing degree. What she lacked in patience, and for that matter in prudence, was more than compensated for by a burning practical charity and selfless devotion to her neighbour that demolished obstacles and enabled her to achieve the impossible with almost monotonous regularity.

Having contracted leoprosy in the course of her work, she was isolated in the primitive leprosarium at Lulindi, isolation being then regarded as the first essential of treatment. The place, a pathetic collection of bamboo huts, was dubbed by its inmates "*Mkaseka*", meaning "Don't laugh [at us]". The primitive conditions did not worry her (she voluntarily lived in similar conditions for the rest of her life) but the iron of segregation, meticulously enforced, ate into her soul, and when eventually she was released as cured, or at least non-infectious, she determined that, if she could help it, no other human being should ever again be so confined.

While in the leprosarium she had been actively engaged in treating her fellow-sufferers, and had selected and trained two of them, Moris and Cuthbert, young men of good education, to assist in this work. As soon as she was released she launched out on a scheme of out-patient clinics, where leprosy could be treated without segregation, the patients living at home and working their fields like their neighbours. She met opposition from her superiors, her fellow-workers and from colonial government officials. Doctors especially said that her scheme was madness, and even decried the treatment she was giving (hydnocarpus oil injections) because it had not been scientifically proved to have a specific effect on the lepra bacillus. As the lepra bacillus would not then grow in captivity, such proof was anyway unattainable. Impatiently she dismissed all such arguments: the patients were getting better, were being cured, and more and more were coming for treatment who had previously hidden themselves away for fear of segregation.

Disparaged and stinted by authority, she used her own money to build and maintain her clinics, and to pay a pittance to her faithful assistants, who stuck to her loyally through thick and thin. As the work grew, calls for help came from ever more distant villages, and she branched out even further, training more workers and building more and bigger clinics.

When I first arrived at Lulindi, Edith Shelley was introduced to me as a very difficult character, and I was warned to be very careful with her. However, I soon came to appreciate what she was doing and the spirit that inspired her work, and was happy to give her all the support I could. In particular I made it my business to integrate her work, until then completely separate, into the general scheme of hospitals and dispensaries. This required some patience and tact, qualities of which I have always been in rather short supply, but eventually it was done, with great advantage all round.

By this time she was working a chain of dispensaries fifty miles long, and travelling between all of them on foot. She lived on the road, and was lucky if she got back to Lulindi once in two weeks. Early in the morning she could be seen setting out before the sun was up, pushing through the long grass drenched with dew, a battered topee on her head and a bulky haversack over her shoulder. Her clothes were the coarsest, home-made and endlessly darned, and her naturally fair skin burnt red like an old tomato. Arrived at a clinic she would open up and sweep out the little hut where she kept a string bed and the bare essentials of life, make herself coffee and scones, and having eaten would bustle around getting the dispensary ready. All day she would be giving injections, and then listening, helping and advising her patients with their problems. Next morning she would be off again to another clinic.

As the work increased, she trained more and more assistants, and divided the area between them. For a time she recruited only ex-patients, feeling that only those who had themselves suffered from leprosy could have the proper approach to the disease.

Presently she could no longer cover the ground efficiently, so she bought a bicycle and extended her work until her furthest clinic was eighty miles from Lulindi, and she was looking still further afield. From then on she was never separated from her bicycle, pedalling it relentlessly through sand and mud, falling into holes, and dragging it uphill, sometimes to the point of complete exhaustion.

In 1939 she developed a cancer. When the diagnosis was confirmed, she demanded that I should "get on and remove it", pointing out that she had previously assisted me in doing such an operation on a patient, so why shouldn't I do it on her? She was with difficulty persuaded to go to England for the operation, where she could receive post-operative X-ray treatment, but made it a condition that she might return immediately it was completed. She went, and was back again in six weeks saying "Well, that's over, I'll never go again!" But she had to admit that she had been overwhelmed by the red-carpet treatment accorded to her at her old hospital in London, where she had innocently supposed that she was forgotten and unloved. Her fame had gone ahead of her.

Back at work, she made the most of her time, but after five years came a generalised recurrence of the cancer and her strength began to fail. She took a long time to die, and as she died she acquired a patience and contentment that were quite new to her. She had never had much time for women, none at all for children or dogs, and in particular had thought very little of our nice young African female nurses (all her assistants were men), but now she began increasingly to appreciate and love them, and in the end would have no one else besides them nursing her.

When she died she had not only cured hundreds, but had won the battle for outpatient treatment and for a saner view of leprosy. Soon afterwards the Colonial Medical Department was loudly advocating (without acknowledgments) the outpatient clinic system throughout Tanganyika.

14

Lulindi Growing, and Ste. Thérèse

The Second World War seemed very remote from Lulindi and life went on much as usual. One difference, however, was that long leave to England was impossible. This proved no hardship, and in fact I found that going quietly on with no prospect of overseas leave had a steadying effect and made for better work. One could plan ahead and carry out one's plans without fear of interruption. However, in 1945, when it was evident that the war was coming to an end, some of us were told to stand by for leave as soon as passages became available. It had been more than seven years since my last leave, so I was to be one of the first to go, but no one had any idea when it would be.

Suddenly the message came. As I emerged from church one Thursday morning, about 6.30 a.m., a messenger handed me a telegram: I was to sail from Dar es Salaam on the Sunday. The road to Masasi was quite impassable for a car, so I had to walk the twenty-four miles. I spent all day clearing up the accumulations of seven years and packing my box. At 5 p.m. I walked out, lamp in hand, my box on the head of a porter. After five miles I stopped at Lusonje to inaugarate a new Scout troop. This was something I had promised to do before I knew I was going, so to keep my promise I enrolled the first new Scouts by lamp-light. Then we sang a few songs and chatted awhile, and I turned in to sleep in the little traveller's hut. I was up and off again before the dawn, and walked into Masasi about 10 a.m. I spent the rest of the day settling affairs at Headquarters, and next morning managed to take a car to Lindi, and thence a flying-boat to Dar es Salaam, arriving just in time to be told that the sailing of the ship was postponed three days.

After a long voyage I arrived in England in time for the annual reunion meeting of the Mission, and stood up to speak for Africa. The hall was packed, with perhaps 2,000 people and with music "like the sound of many waters" they sang the mission hymn:

Fling out the banner! Let it float,
Skyward and seaward, high and wide—
The sun that lights its shining folds
The Cross on which our Saviour died.

The atmosphere was deeply emotional, yet completely sane. Africa was calling to England, and at least a part of England wanted to hear. When I stood up, there was an intense silence of expectation. I had been in the bush for ten years, and was no longer a novice. In the plainest simplest words I drew a picture of Africa and the poverty of our medical service.

I let them imagine the map of Tanganyika superimposed on the map of England. We were meeting in Westminster: "Let this represent Tandahimba, a place with a big population and a boarding school, but still no dispensary even. Suppose you live here and your child is sick, the nearest dispensary is at Coulsdon (Nanyamba) or near to Hatfield (Mahuta), whichever you prefer, but nothing nearer, and to get there you must walk and carry your child: there is no public transport. Even then, there is no doctor at either. If you want to see a doctor (me!) you must walk on nearly to Cambridge (Lulindi). Even then, you will have to pay a small fee. If, as a taxpayer, you want to claim a free consultation from the nearest Government doctor, you must walk to Eastbourne (Mikindani). My brothers and sisters, we *must* at least put a dispensary at Tandahimba, and many other places too." The audience were appalled, and they gave generously.

I spent my leave collecting funds and equipment, and recruiting new workers, notably Ronald Heald, a male nurse of tremendous character who carried on where Edith Shelley had left off, and battled with leprosy day and night for more than twenty-five years.

With various gifts and legacies I was able on my return to expand Lulindi hospital, building additional wards and a new operating theatre, X-ray, and maternity block. I was tired of thatched roofs, with all their disadvantages and dangers (their one big advantage is heat insulation), and determined to try tiling the hospital. Corrugated iron, the universal East African roof, is expensive, hot, noisy and unattractive. There was good potters' clay at Lulindi, which should be good for tiles, but no one locally knew how to make them. I therefore sent off two of the Scouts, Viktor Mangame and Luka Ausi, to Msumba on the shores of Lake Nyasa to learn the art. On their return they taught other Scouts, and we soon had a big output of attractive pantiles in the Italian style. Life was not too easy, however. We chose the driest part of the year for our tile-making, but a quite unseasonable deluge of rain ruined several thousand tiles that were drying on the ground and caused our beautiful bee-hive kiln to collapse with as many more inside it. We eventually had a large part of the hospital roofed with nice red tiles but a year later they all began quietly to disintegrate! That was the end of tiles in Lulindi.

Among the new equipment the most exciting was a semi-portable X-ray machine—semi-portable for the sake of economy. After working in the dark for more than ten years the relief of being able to visualise fractures and foreign bodies, at least, was tremendous. Bess Grant, who came as our radiographer, was another great character, and a wonderful asset.

An X-ray machine of course meant an electric generator, and so at last we could have electric light. After years of wrestling with oil lamps and electric torches it was marvellous to be able to switch on, at least for night emergencies. We had no scyalitic lamp for the theatre, so we made do with the scheme used at the London Hospital in Theatres 1-5 for more than forty years, namely two 500-watt lamps placed three feet apart over the table with big reflectors. This throws a flood of light on to the table, each lamp lighting up the shadows cast by the other. Rigby, Sherren, Walton, Lett and Souttar had no other lighting in their day, so why should we worry? It worked beautifully, and was a great comfort when dealing with the frightful sort of emergencies that so often seemed to come in the middle of the night.

Once in Lulindi, in the depth of the rains, the Matron became seriously ill. She appeared to be developing septicaemia and was getting worse. Penicillin was still a new wonder and we had none, but it looked as if the Matron might die unless I could find some.

We knew there was penicillin in the outside world, but where? Possibly Masasi, more probably Ndanda or Lindi, but how could we get there in time? The whole world (our world) was waterlogged and we had not attempted motoring for some months. But to walk on such an uncertain errand, twenty-five or fifty miles and back again was too slow. Desperate measures were called for, so I set out in the ambulance at 6 a.m. to see how far I could go. We wallowed through mud and water for fourteen miles, surprisingly well, and then came to the first big obstacle, the Mwiti river. The bridge had been completely washed away and the water had spread some distance over the banks on both sides. The river was not very deep and the bottom was sandy. I had halted close by to plan a possible crossing when I suddenly heard the improbable sound of a motor engine roaring and the shouts, cheers and singing of a great crowd of men. Incredibly somebody was fording the river. I ran down to the bank and saw to my amazement a large pick-up, obviously heavily loaded, in midstream and well awash, being pushed and pulled by the entire riverside population. The car was an unfamiliar one (we knew all the local vehicles) and how any stranger had ever reached that point from Masasi was unimaginable.

Eventually the amphibian came up on to dry ground and stopped. A red-faced smiling figure stepped out and said "Good morning, I am Dr. Eckhart, I have come from Arusha and I am going to Mtwara to be the first doctor to cope with the new groundnut port." I asked if he was alone. He was, but he said that he had all his equipment in the car. Had he any penicillin? "Yes, as much as you want, but have you any cash? Mine is all finished!" That was easy—I gave him cash, and he gave me a large box of penicillin, and by 8 a.m. I was back at Lulindi, and injected the Matron with penicillin. She got better.

About this time Lulindi happened to be chosen as the place for the annual diocesan retreat; as it was holiday time, the buildings of the girls' schools, up a hill about half a mile from the hospital, were used. This made it possible for me to attend the retreat while still on call for the hospital in emergency. During the retreat I read, by way of recreation, the life of St. Thérèse of Lisieux. I found it fascinating, especially the account of her posthumous miracles—the "shower of roses"— but a friend said "That's a dangerous book. She'll lead you to Rome!" Meanwhile, in the middle of the retreat, I was suddenly called to the hospital, and found a child who had been brought in choking. I saw at once that he had a huge retropharyngeal abscess and was dying of asphyxia. He was already deeply cyanotic and unconscious, his breath coming in failing gasps. I said "Nurse, hold him upside down quick!" and seizing the nearest instrument, I punctured the abscess. A river of pus flowed out, but at that very moment the failing respiration stopped altogether. The child went limp, and looked utterly dead. I had seen this happen twice before in bush practice, where hours of unrelieved asphyxia finally damage the brain beyond recovery from lack of oxygen, and resuscitation is useless. But this time I had a new weapon. Desperately I called on St. Thérèse "Pray for this child!" Immediately, breathing began again, quite and regular. The child made a good recovery, and I went back to my retreat. St. Thérèse has been my friend ever since.

Besides the development of the hospital, the dispensaries and the leprosy clinics, two other activities were growing apace. One was the Nursing School which from small beginnings was slowly but surely turning out increasing numbers of dependable fully-trained nurses. At the very beginning Miss Bell had insisted that we must set the highest standards, and had based her syllabus on the British model in such a way that the students were taught everything possible within our limited facilities, with room to expand whenever opportunity allowed. This produced excellent results, with emphasis on the compassionate care of the sick.

Of all the work in which I have been privileged to take part, none has been more rewarding than the training of Tanzanian nurses, and seeing them take, without wavering, the heavy responsibilities that fall on a ward sister or staff-nurse in a one-doctor hospital, with corresponding lightening of the doctor's load. I still remember the casual remark of our matron: "You know, our patients really are being nursed." It was a remark that was echoed over the years at both my later hospitals, and heartened me immensely. It was reflected in the habit of our student-nurses' often starting an urgent report to me with the words: "My patient. . ."

It is strange that two nurses who in later years proved to be among the most capable and reliable I have known should have been, as students, men whom I was on the point of throwing out as hopeless. This only shows that vocation is more important than formal training. In 1948 one of our finalists, now Mrs. Sarah Nyirenda, became the first Tanganyikan nurse to win the territorial silver medal (there is no gold medal). Our syllabus was adopted by the Government and began to be used all over the country as new schools grew up and more and more nurses were trained.

A day was to come more than twenty years later when Government was so ill advised as to propose the removal of more than 1,000 Tanzanian nurses from the Register as they were considered not quite internationally respectable. I had by then become an M.P., so, knowing the calibre of our nurses, I immediately attacked the Bill in Parliament. I spoke from the heart, and soon Members were running into the house to defend Tanzania's nurses against a measure of unimaginative bureaucracy. After about an hour of this, an embarrassed Minister withdrew the Bill, and it has never been heard of again.

As well as the nursing students, I also had a group of learner-dressers, who lived with me in a small hostel and learned what they could on the job. They had no formal course of instruction, but they were bright boys and quick to learn, and mostly very keen.

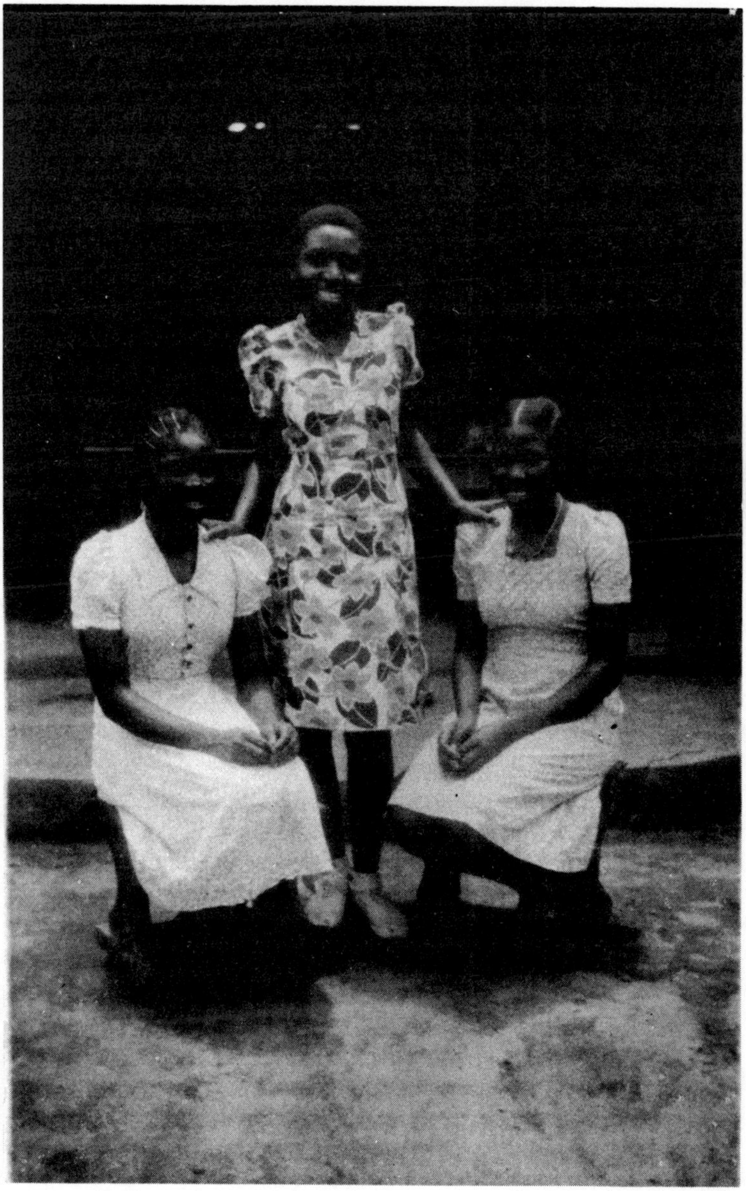

Lulindi nurses off duty. The Author's future wife is on the right, and the Silver Medallist in the centre.

Moris was rather too bright. He had an excitable and volatile temperament and was always doing something unexpected and often disconcerting, even if it was only emitting peals of near-hysterical laughter or having a fight about nothing. One day he got hold of a bunch of bananas, which had been set aside for staff refreshment, and carefully injected each banana with a hypodermic syringe filled with quinine. The result can be imagined, but it took no time to detect the perpetrator. No one else would have thought of such a trick, and anyway he was laughing his head off. The laugh was duly transferred to "the other side of his face" by his infuriated companions.

The other activity was Scouting, which had quickly covered almost the whole of the vast neglected Southern Province of Tanganyika, for which I held a Commissioner's warrant. In 1947 the first ever East African Jamboree was held near Kampala in Uganda, and in a Tanganyika contingent of 120 picked Scouts the Southern Province was able to contribute fifty. We assembled at Masasi and travelled by open lorry three days through the forest to Dar es Salaam, camping each night, then two days by train to Mwanza, and finally two days by steamer across Lake Victoria, altogether about 1,400 miles. Our scouts camped for a week in a strange land and covered themselves with glory for their smartness, their traditional dancing and their first-aid display, in which they rescued a helpless man from a fiercely blazing hut, the victim being carried out on his camp-bed in flames. We had devised a way of having the bed clothes ablaze without burning the patient, so it made a great sensation. On the return journey we met a leopard, elephants and all kinds of wild beasts, but arrived home intact, and singing loudly. We returned on a Friday which in those days was still a day of abstinence, but the Bishop dispensed the Scout movement for the occasion so that we could feast, and we did.

In 1948 I was appointed Commissioner for Training and spent the next fifteen years building up the training team and organising training courses for Scoutmasters, at various levels, to cover the whole of Tanganyika. This fascinating work was even more rewarding than running Scout troops.

It was about this time that at our rallies and training courses we began to sing "God bless Africa", the song of African independence. It had come up from South Africa, and had been translated into several East African languages. Probably the Scouts of Bukoba, in the extreme north-west, got it first, but after the East

African Jamboree it rapidly spread everywhere. The tune is deeply moving and fourteen years later it was adopted as the National Anthem of Tanganyika. Some of the stuffier imperialist types were shocked, but we went on singing it.

15

"On this Rock", and my Second Hospital

Life is made up of problems, and while all this happy activity was going on, a big problem was smouldering away just under the surface. It finally erupted in 1949 and ended my fourteen years of service with the Universities' Mission. I had joined the Church of England as a student, under the influence of some of my friends, but I had already learned the Catholic faith at the age of ten, and had always tacitly accepted it as the real thing. In Africa I had found the Catholic Church everywhere, always pressing forward to new frontiers, fulfilling its divine mission of "preaching the Gospel to every creature". To offer to Africa the fruits of the European reformation, in obvious competition with "the faith once delivered to the Saints", seemed to me an unwarranted impertinence, and as the years passed I found the situation becoming increasingly intolerable. Already in 1946 I had discussed this with the Bishop (Bishop L. E. Stradling, later of Johnnesburg), and found him understanding and sympathetic, but what was to be done? All that we had been building up, with sweat and prayer, day after day and year after year, and the faith of our African brothers were things too precious to be lightly jettisoned.

Eventually in 1947 I composed a letter to the Bishop drawing his attention to the scandal of disunity in presenting the Gospel to Africa, and the urgency of reunion. I begged him to consult with his fellow-bishops with a view to a corporate approach to the Holy See. I circulated this letter to the other members of the Mission in the Diocese and obtained the ready signatures of all but one of the clergy and half the laity. Thus fortified I presented the letter to the Bishop. He accepted it, and put it before the other three Bishops of the Universities' Mission. They in turn endorsed it and sent it to the Archbishop of Canterbury at Lambeth. There it seems to have raised some eyebrows, but it was adroitly passed to the Church of England's Foreign Relations Committee (this seemed to me an amusing touch) who shelved it to await the Lambeth Conference of 1948. As this was about as much as we could expect, we the signatories to the letter sat back and waited. I continued to pray "Thy Kingdom Come" and to repair hernias and wild-beast injuries as usual.

The 1948 Lambeth Conference came and went. There were no headlines on re-union. Eventually one of our number, meeting a bishop in the street, asked him what had happened to our plea. The bishop replied that there had been so many urgent matters that they had never got round to it. So the reunion of the sundered body of Christ was not a matter of the first urgency! It was time to stand up and be counted, and six of us, after some desperate last-minute attempts to find a way of corporate reunion, accepted the simple words of the Gospel for what they have always been: "Thou art Peter, and on this rock I will build my Church." We made our ways individually as best we could. Another fifteen former members of the Mission and mission workers followed later. The adventures of two of the Sisters would be hardly credible nowadays, but they made it. For myself, I was conveniently due for leave.

Nowadays, the relations between the Catholic and Anglican Churches in Southern Tanzania are remarkable for their harmony and practical cooperation, but in those pre-ecumenical days it was unthinkable to have a non-Anglican doctor working in an Anglican hospital, so I simply handed my resignation to the Bishop, with profound regrets, and packed my boxes for the last time, working in the hospital to the end. On the last morning I went along to hospital prayers as usual and then said a short farewell. "I am following Unity", I said. It was difficult to say much more without hurting someone. Then the staff sang "God be with you till we meet again" and began to cry. I fled.

I went first to Ndanda, where the sons of St. Benedict took me in their arms, and next day passed me on to their brothers at Dar es Salaam. Ten days later, on Easter morning, I made my peace with the Catholic Church.

The Abbot-Bishop of Ndanda, the late Mgr. Viktor Haelg, O.S.B., accepted me for work forthwith, and on my return from leave I was sent to a remote mission in the Mwera country called Mnero, with instructions, once again, to build up a hospital. It was a well established mission, with a lovely church and the usual fruits of Benedictine industry in gardens, farm and workshops. Medically however, there was only a small dispensary, which did not even have running water, although water was laid on everywhere else, even in the cow-byre! The Father Superior, the late Dom Columban Furrer, was a Swiss, very gentle and made me very much at home. I made a quick tour of the outlying dispensaries for which I would have to be responsible, and then settled down to build the hospital. That is to say, I drew rough plans, but this time I was provided with a real architect, Brother Adelhard Pfisterer, O.S.B., who translated them into something that would not easily fall down, and then stayed to supervise the building.

Long before the hospital was completed, the Bishop ordered me to open a school for male nurses. This was highly congenial, but to start the school without buildings or equipment was a strain on everybody. We borrowed a disused classroom for our lessons, and the students slept and ate in a small mud hut previously used for casual baptismal candidates. Practical work was done in the barn-like buildings in which the dispensary patients lodged. One of them had no windows at all and was promptly called by the students "the black hole". They were very cheerful and keen to learn, but they were only promoted dressers and their lack of education made progress hard. The Sister Tutor was the Matron of Ndanda hospital fifty miles away, and so could only come and teach once a month. For the rest of the time most of the teaching, apart from my own, was given by a very able Medical Assistant, Leo Ibihya. He was tall and very thin, and always looked rather as though he had been washed and hung out to dry. He had a rare gift for teaching, and was so keen that he laid a really solid foundation in anatomy, physiology, hygiene, and nursing. He rarely had any failures among students. In the end only one student of the first intake withdrew, and all the rest passed their finals. Most of them are holding responsible positions to this day. Our next intake were of better higher education, and the results even better, our Senior Student, Daniel G. Mkwela, winning the Tanganyika silver medal in the final examination.

The building of the hospital went on too slowly, so the students and I lent a hand whenever we had finished our medical work. We helped with the roofing (as I had so often done at Lulindi) and went far out into the forest to haul timber, first on our shoulders, then precariously on a handcart, and finally towing behind a car.

While the building continued, the numbers of patients were increasing, and their cases had to be dealt with in whatever space was available. When an operation was needed I could either do it in the very small pharmacy (eight feet square and full of bottles) or else turn all the patients out of the outpatient room and do it there.

Neither site was ideal, but I managed to cope with what came, including two cases of cerebral compression from extradural abscess. Less urgent major cases I transferred when possible to Ndanda, and operated in their excellent theatre there.

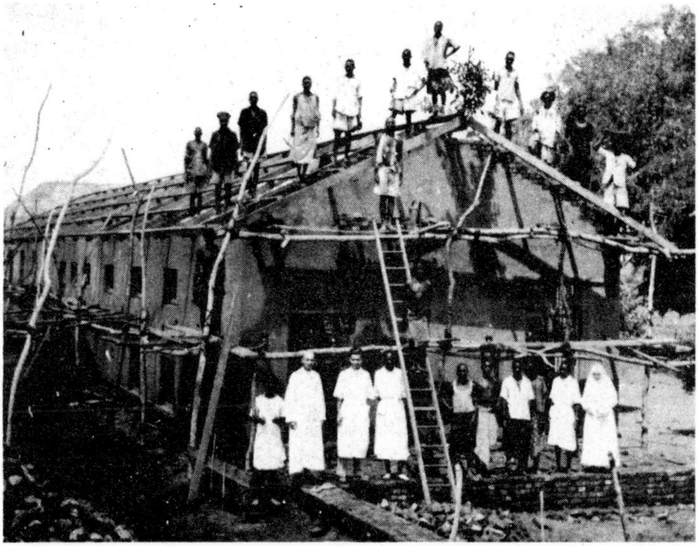

Above, building Mnero Hospital. Standing, to left of ladder (l. to r.): Dom Tassilo Jaeger, the Author, Leo Ibihya. *Below*, a ward verandah at Mnero.

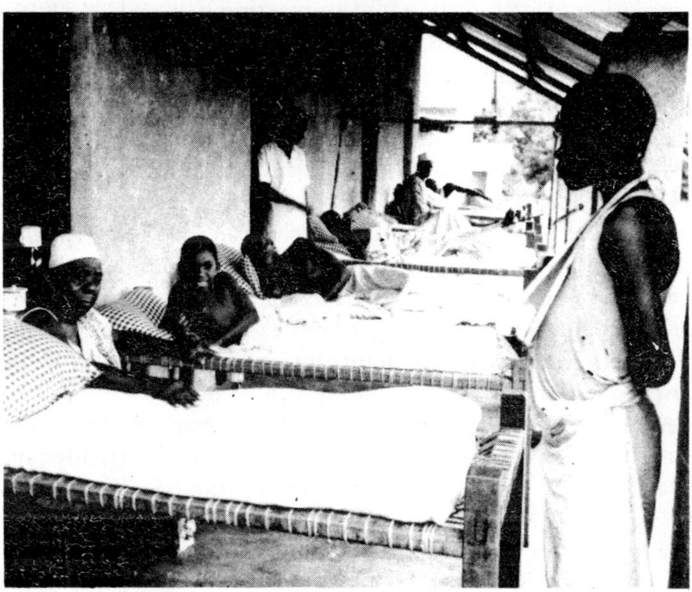

One day when visiting a remote dispensary I saw a young man walking around quite fit, smiling and gesticulating. They said he could not speak, since a week before when he had been hit on the head in a fight. I put my hand to the left side of his head, and at once felt a sharp depression in the skull. I said he should come to hospital for an operation, and rather to my surprise he agreed, so to Ndanda we went. I operated with local anaesthesia as usual, and I had no sooner raised the depressed piece of bone than a sepulchral voice from under the sterile drapes said "Doctor, I hold your feet!" the usual greeting to one's elders. He went home talking volubly and everyone was happy.

The building as usual had all to be done from scratch. Bricks were fired on the spot and doors and windows made in the mission carpenters' shop from local timber. For roofing this time I used corrugated aluminium, which is lighter and cooler than corrugated iron. The general plan was the same as Lulindi, compact to save the feet of the limited staff, but with plenty of light and air. The wards had wide verandahs and all the beds strong wheels, so that patients could be wheeled out as soon as they had had their morning treatment, and spend the rest of the day on the verandah; there they could be visited by their relatives without restriction of hours. Meanwhile the ward could be washed down and swept thoroughly while the patients were outside, thereby minimising cross-infection and preventing dirt and smells in the ward. At sunset the beds were all wheeled in again, a very simple procedure. At night there was still no lack of ventilation; although the doors and windows were securely shut, the wards had no ceilings, and so air could circulate freely from under the eaves.

We managed to obtain a good X-ray machine (the same model as Lulindi) and so once more we could use the generator to light the hospital. I also installed an internal telephone (the nearest external one was still twenty miles away). The great groundnut scheme was in the process of collapsing and I was able to buy twenty telephones for ten shillings each. Having a bedside telephone, and so able to talk intelligently with the night-duty nurse, I was saved many a time from the necessity of getting out of bed.

A curiosity of our telephones was that apparently they did not understand Swahili. Although my students normally spoke Swahili, whenever two of them were on the telephone together they spoke to each other in the most careful English.

While all this building was going on, I was suddenly attacked by the Government Medical Department on the ground that the facilities provided by the hospital were inadequate for the proper training of nurses. This was perfectly true, but we were in fact managing quite well in spite of everything, and the morale of the students was high—nor could I let down the Bishop who had landed me in an impossible position. I therefore had to exert all my diplomacy in a long drawn-out correspondence with distant Dar es Salaam while the facilities provided were being stepped up as fast as possible. It was all quite reprehensible, but knowing some of the tricks which the colonial Government had themselves got up to, and got away with, I was not worried. Eventually we were visited by a representative of the Director of Medical Services. I had known this man in student days; indeed the last time I remembered seeing him, he was being forcibly restrained from running naked down the Victoria Embankment in London late one night. Naturally we did not discuss the episode, but I have the feeling it was in the back of his mind. He was very affable, and all passed off well.

As soon as the hospital was built, I insisted on proper accommodation for my students. The primary school had just been moved to new premises, so we took over their good two-storey building close to the hospital, which we renovated and extended. It made a pleasant nurses' hostel. I moved out of the Benedicitine monastry and occupied a room on the first floor of the hostel, so that I was with my students. Formal classes were held in the hospital, where I had equipped a lecture and practice room and a teaching laboratory, but in the evenings in the hostel, after eating and praying together, we had discussions, debates, plays and informal instruction on many things, with guest speakers whenever possible. The students also danced rumbas (all male!) and sang a lot. They were very lively, and in the afternoons whoever was free did some scouting, ran a football team, cultivated gardens or played badminton. It was a happy family.

One of the innovations in building the hospital and the students' hostel was water-borne sanitation. This was still something new in Southern Tanganyika, and during all the years at Lulindi we had none. Having ample piped water at Mnero (from an excellent well that tapped the underground Mnero river) it was an obvious step to install shower-baths and water-closets. However, to people who had never seen a water-closet it presented certain problems. Especially they had to learn that it was not an oubliette for any old rubbish such as corn-cobs and banana-skins, which rapidly brought the system to an embarrassing standstill.

The students, of course, were in a position to learn these points more rapidly than the patients. Even so, after some time the hostel drains showed signs of total obstruction. Simple methods of relief having failed, there was nothing for it but to open up the whole system, so after dark I assembled the whole school and pointed out that as obviously some of them had caused the obstruction, it was up to them to relieve it. I gave them tools and rigged a large electric light from the bathroom window, and the students, suitably clad or rather un-clad, began to open up the drain. It was not a pleasant job, but they worked light-heartedly with a lot of banter. About 10 o'clock there was a sudden shout of triumph as a filthy and at first unrecognisable object was extracted from the hole and the blockage was at once released. Someone held it up on stick: a pair of shorts! There was a roar of shouting and laughter, and then much ribald speculation as to how the shorts had got there and to whom they belonged. Their owner never revealed himself—anyway, it never happened again.

In 1959 we changed from male-nurse training to training rural medical aids in order to staff the rural dispensaries where the need was more acute than in the hospitals. The basis of the training was the same, and life in the hostel went on as before. As we were then the only training school in Tanganyika for rural medical aids, apart from the one Government school at Mwanza, we were drawing students from all over the country, which added interest and broadened the outlook of everyone. Of course, most of the students returned to their own areas when they qualified, so they are now to be found working all over Tanzania. Many of them have done further training and been upgraded to become medical assistants. In recent years the school has been moved to Masasi, where I first began, and it now has even finer buildings and equipment, a larger intake of students and is doing a great work. But their chief instructor is still an old Mnero student

One special difficulty at Mnero was a strong local taboo against being carried on a bed or hammock. This had been the usual mode of transport for stretcher-cases at Lulindi, and in fact we kept two hammocks on poles which could be borrowed to bring patients in to the hospital, the paths being mostly impassable for a wheeled ambulance. The Wamwera, however, regarded being carried on a bed as the privilege of a corpse, and absolutely refused to be carried while still alive, being certain that this was asking for death. This led to the extraordinary practice of bringing in patients with acute pneumonia, or women in labour, on the carrier of a bicycle. If there was no bicycle, the patient just died at home.

Otherwise, medical problems at Mnero and its dispensaries were much the same as at Lulindi, but they were never lacking in variety, and all too often had an element of tragedy. One evening after dark a young woman stood in the open doorway of her hut, the fire burning behind her and her baby at her breast. Suddenly a leopard sprang out of the darkness, grabbed the baby and knocked the woman backwards on to the fire. The men of the village pursued the leopard, and eventually retrieved the head and shoulders of the baby: the leopard had eaten the rest. This piece they then used to bait a trap for the leopard. In the morning they brought the woman to hospital with severe burns and distraught from the loss of her child. She made a good recovery from the burns, but there was nothing we could do about the baby, and they even failed to trap the leopard.

On another occasion a man arrived at Nyangao dispensary on his hands and knees, having only one foot. He had crawled like this about fifteen miles, and when I asked where his other foot was, he said it had dropped off in the road. This was apparently a case of gangrene from a puff-adder bite. Puff-adders are the commonest poisonous snakes in the country around Masasi and Mnero, and although their bite rarely kills it can cause the loss of a foot or part of a leg. I found, however, that these cases respond well to simple surgical principles (elevation of the leg with absolute rest, incision and hypertonic compresses, antibiotics, vasodilators and morphia) and with this regime I had never seen gangrene develop. It develops readily enough, however, in those who walk about looking for anti-snake medicine. There are many local remedies for snakebite, their chief aim being to make the victim vomit. From the pathology of snake-bite it is highly improbable that any of them has any useful effect, the high recovery rate being due to the non-poisonous character of most local snakes. Apart from puff-adders, the two commonest poisonous snakes are the cobra and the mamba (green or black according to age). The cobra usually contents itself with spitting, and if the venom enters an eye it is extremely painful, though the sight can be saved. If it does bite, it is serious. The only occasion on which I was able to use snake anti-venom successfully was when a man was biten by a cobra one night close to the hospital, and was admitted after only a few minutes. He had severe pain, and already had constriction of his chest and throat with distressed breathing and failing pulse. I gave him 40 c.c. of anti-venom promptly and he recovered. Usually by the time a snakebite patient reaches hospital it is already too late for anti-venom, or more often, the bite was not serious and so there is no need for it. Mamba bites are not common, but they are so bad that the patient never reaches hospital alive. Almost the only hope would be to have advance warning that a snake was going to bite, and to be standing ready with a syringe loaded with the special anti-mamba serum!

Snakes are naturally a source of great dread, especially as most people are very vague about the different species and cannot distinguish the few really poisonous ones. In any case, snakes tend to go about at night, and in the dark it is difficult to know what sort it is. The first case of snakebite I ever had to deal with was in a young woman who had been gathering firewood. She was brought into Lulindi in a state of terror, especially as the snake had escaped alive, this being regarded as a very bad omen. I examined her carefully and could find no signs of anything wrong, no swelling, no paralysis, no change in pulse or respiration. I concluded that the snake had been a non-poisonous one, and tried to reassure her. Nothing any of us could do had any effect. She screamed and screamed, saying she was going to die, and after about nine hours she did. There was no sign of poisoning right up to the end, and I am sure she died of fright. Until then I had not believed this to be possible. If I had, I would have put her out with a hypnotic injection (intramuscular hexobarbitone is the easiest, most effective and longest-acting, though seldom used nowadays; we had no largactil in those days) and kept her unconsious long enough to obliterate her terror. I have often regretted bitterly that I did not do so, but I simply could not believe that she could die. We learn at other people's expense.

Of numerous personal meetings with snakes I vividly remember three. The first was a green mamba, yards of it and brilliant green, draped casually across the path from one bush to another like a Christmas decoration. The bush was dense, and there was no way round; the snake showed no sign of moving. There seemed nothing else to do, so I simply ducked underneath with the feeling of a child playing "Oranges and Lemons". When I turned back to have another look, the snake had gone, so presumably it was not asleep after all. Had I known then (it was in my early days) exactly how deadly the mamba is, I think I would have sat down to wait!

On the second occasion I was walking briskly along a stony path through the forest. There were dead branches of trees lying about, and I did just notice a long grey piece of dry wood lying along the edge of the path. As I passed it my boot struck a stone rather sharply, and the piece of wood suddenly leapt in the air and went roaring off through the dry forest. It was a huge grey cobra, and went at lightning speed with its head carried high, at least two feet off the ground, and its neck full-expanded. It was a terrifying sight, but I think it was as startled as I (it had probably been asleep), and at least it rushed *away* from me.

Not so the third one. I was sitting, privately as I thought, on a pit latrine, when a snake suddenly rushed in through the open doorway and dived between my legs and down the hole. I had no time to do anything, but the snake completely ignored me. I suppose it was coming home!

For various technical reasons, most of the surgery done in Southern Tanzania, apart from a few "head and neck" cases, is what is usually known as "subumbilical". The male cases include a number of conditions known collectively as "*mshipa*", literally "a sinew" but actually a euphemism for any sort of scrotal swelling. Many of these were hernias, some of enormous size. The biggest I ever met hung down to the patient's knees. Although a left-sided hernia it contained the caecum and appendix (from the right side) as well as the transverse and pelvic colon and in fact most of what he'd got. The chief difficulty was to get all the guts back into his belly, from which they had been so long absent, but in the end I succeeded.

Among the biggest swellings were many cases of elephantiasis, a horrible affliction due to filarial worms carried by a mosquito. Although it is never seen in England, I found several operations for it described in English books. They proved far from satisfactory, being both mutilating and bloody, so I developed my own operation, which was designed to minimise bleeding and to finish up with a plastic reconstruction giving a nice cosmetic result. I never wrote it up, but was gratified to discover many years later that it had been adopted as far away as Kampala in Uganda. For the very big masses I devised a sterilised crane with which to manoeuvre them. There is a picture in the books of a man with an elephantoid mass weighing more than 200 lb., but I never met one so large. The heaviest I have removed weighed 40 lb., which is quite heavy enough to have hanging between your legs, and throwing you off your balance as you attempt to walk. That patient came from about a hundred miles away, through the bush, so I asked him how he had managed it. "Well", he said, "I walked a little and I rested a little. Then I walked a little and I rested a little, until I got here." One hundred miles! I have no adequate comment.

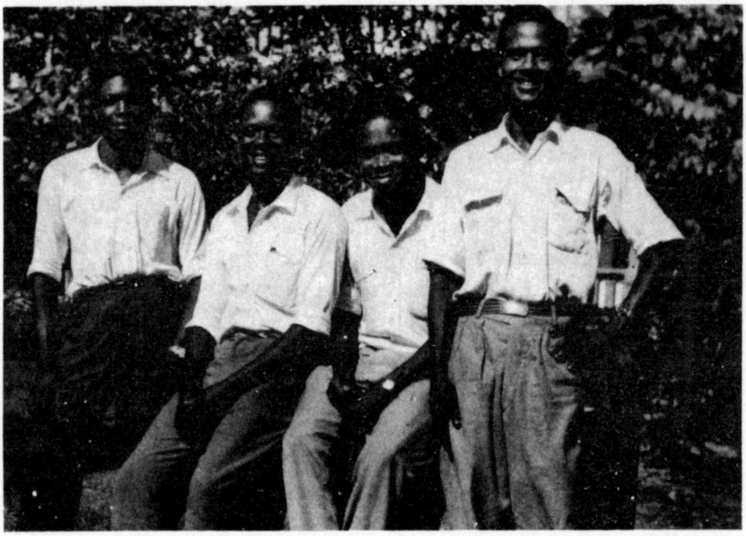

A group of students at Mnero.

16
More Scouting

I had only been at Mnero a week when three small boys stood in front of me and asked, innocently but directly, "When are you going to start the Scouts?" My heart sank. I thought I had started enough scout troops in my time, and that the job of Territorial Training Commissioner was quite enough. Besides, I had to concentrate on building a hospital and starting a nursing school. However, there was no escape, and so we began all over again, on the same lines as at Lulindi, and soon had a very happy troop running. It drew candidates from the primary school, from the nursing school and from no school at all, so it was healthily mixed and quite independent.

As at Lulindi the Father Superior was at first suspicious of our activities, but before long he became an enthusiastic supporter, and called on the Scouts to undertake many responsible duties.

Our activities gradually grew more ambitious than at Lulindi, and we carried out ever larger "pioneering" projects, with some climbing and camping in several nice rocky hills round about. Our pioneering was not merely ornamental, as we were asked by the District Commissioner to build a permanent footbridge over a seasonal torrent that cut off a school and a village, and when the Mnero Valley was flooded we made a large raft with the idea of ferrying prople over, there being no other way across. Our raft was strong but the current was stronger, and on our first trip we were carried away and disappeared quickly downstream. The news immediately spread that the doctor was drowned, though it was taken very calmly. However, no one came to any harm. When we could no longer control our headlong course with our poles we dropped off into the water and swam the raft ashore.

The Mnero Scouts were certainly adventurous, and decided there was no reason why camping should be restricted, as it always was, to the dry season. Two of the Senior Scouts wanted to do a test hike, so although it was the middle of the rainy season they were determined to spend the night on the top of Ndangalimbo, one of our rocky hills a few miles away. They set out after mid-day and their patrol leader and I promised to visit them later in the day to see how they were getting on. We took a jeep near to the foot of the hill, and then climbed. On reaching the summit we found they had securely pitched their tent, anchoring it with stones, and had made a fine fire under the lee of a great overhanging rock. The

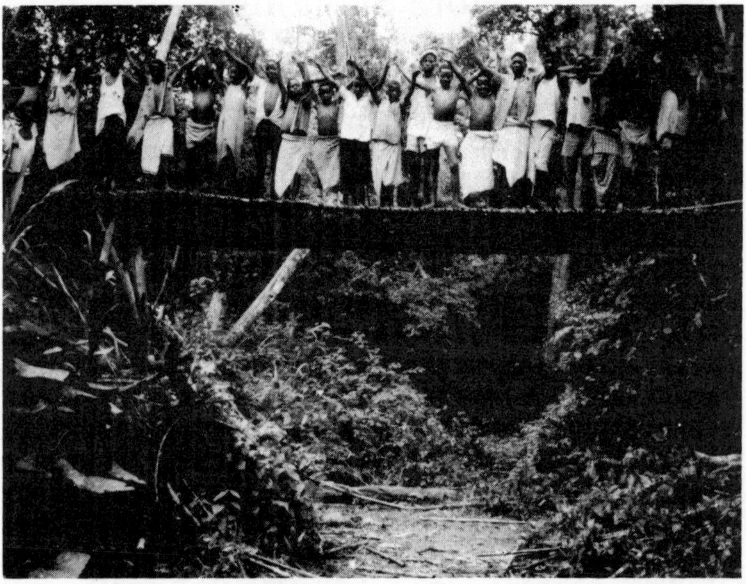

Above, bridge built by Mnero Scouts—with the builders. *Below,* first aid practice—Mnero Scouts. (Photo: Benedictine Abbey, Ndanda.)

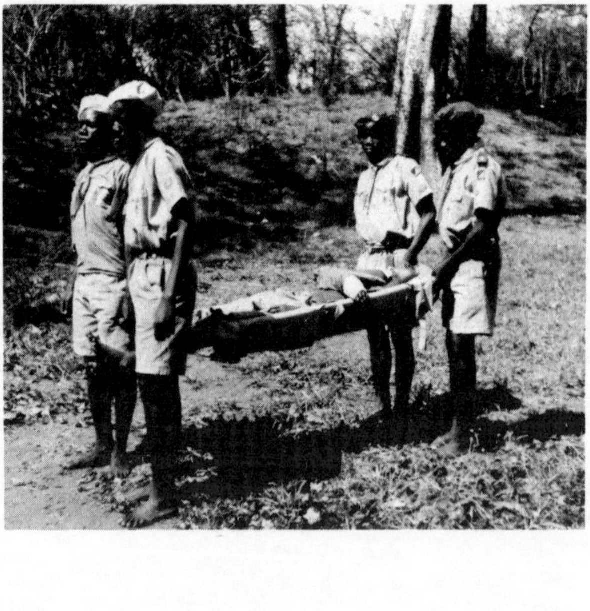

cook was already preparing supper and they seemed well set and in good form. Suddenly someone said "Look at that!" "That" was a black wall of solid rain sweeping straight at us from the valley. We dived into the tent and it hit us like a bomb. In a few moments the world was a swirling flood in inky darkness. The water poured in under the uphill end of the tent (it was pitched on a slight slope) and went rushing out at the door. We hastily scooped out a channel for it and then sat on the banks on either side and watched it swirl by in the lamplight. I put on a mac and ventured out to see how the cook was faring, but his shelter was good and his fire roared. He soon had supper cooked, and we scrambled back into the tent and made a good meal, still on the banks of our little river.

Eventually the rain eased off, so the Patrol Leader and I pulled on our macs and wished the adventurous pair a good night. We set off down the familiar path by the light of an electric torch. At first all went well; from the peak we came down on to a long ridge, but then we had to find the point at which to leave the ridge and drop down to the plain. In dry weather and by daylight this was easy enough, but on a pitch dark night in pouring rain and amid the dense overgrown vegetation of the rainy season it was not. We stumbled back and forth and up and down, scrambling over rocks we had never noticed before, and falling into chasms, all in the dark, until we were tired and wet and completely lost. Well, not quite completely, as the ridge ran east and west, and was quite straight and fairly narrow, so we had a base-line, but we could not find the patch down the north side of the ridge, and without the path descent was impossible, as the ground was far too broken and there were dense woods at the bottom. Our only way was to scramble down the south side of the ridge, which was steeper and had no path at all, but it was easier going and we knew there was a well-worn path at the bottom running along the foot of the hill, which we could not miss. However, to get down even there in pitch darkness was impractical, so we decided to wait for the moon to rise, which we reckoned would be about midnight. It was now only 10 p.m., so we settled down on a great wet slab of rock, pulled our hoods well over and huddled together for warmth. And still the rain came down.

At midnight, sure enough, the moon rose but the clouds were so heavy that it gave only a pale glimmer through the trees and we had to wait another hour until it was high enough to give us any light. Then at last we set off, wet, cold and cramped, and with our torch and the moon we slithered and scrambled down the steep hillside, through dense bushes and jungle grass and over and under rocks until at last we reached the bottom. There was no difficulty in finding the path, and with great relief we strode smartly round the base of the hill. We soon found the jeep, clambered in and set off. The rain had at last stopped, and we were speeding happily along when we came suddenly on the Mnero river, which had once more flooded after the night's torrential rain and was totally impassible. It was now 3 a.m., so we simply curled up in the jeep and slept the best we could.

At dawn we surveyed the flood. It was going down, and there was no more rain, but it would be several hours before even a jeep could cross, so the Patrol Leader, being a student-nurse and due to go on duty at 7 a.m., waded through the waist-deep flood and set off for home, while I waited to rescue the jeep when I could. By 8 a.m., the water was only knee-deep, so I coaxed the jeep through and was soon home. The two Scouts on test returned in good order later in the day, so all ended well, but the Father Superior—then Dom Tassilo Jaeger, O.S.B.—said he had never heard of anything so completely stupid!

In 1952 there was another Jamboree, held in what was then Northern Rhodesia and is now Zambia, to which I led a contingent of ninety Tanganyikan Scouts. Our contingent as usual was multiracial, but having heard that there was a strong colour-bar in Northern Rhodesia, we deliberately made up a mixed patrol, African, Indian, European, and half-caste, who camped together very happily and were an object of wonder to local Rhodesians who came in crowds to see them. Again we won fame for our displays of songs and dances, and another sensational first-aid stunt in which some initial clowning led to incipient tragedy, and a snake-bite victim (Amadeo, an amazingly agile climber) was lowered by rope from a seventy-five-foot tree. The suspense was good, and had the colonial Governor and all the VIPs on their feet. We made rather a point of these sensational stunts, as I found the conventional first-aid displays terribly dull and unconvincing. In one of our most successful stunts at another rally we completely ran over a boy with a Land Rover and then patched him up and carried him off on an improvised stretcher. It was almost *too* good, as some of the local elders said "That boy really was killed, but the Scouts revived him with their 'medicine'", this carrying a possible implication of witchcraft, which I did not care for!

Our scouts not only took many songs with them but at the Jamboree collected many more. On our return the dispersing

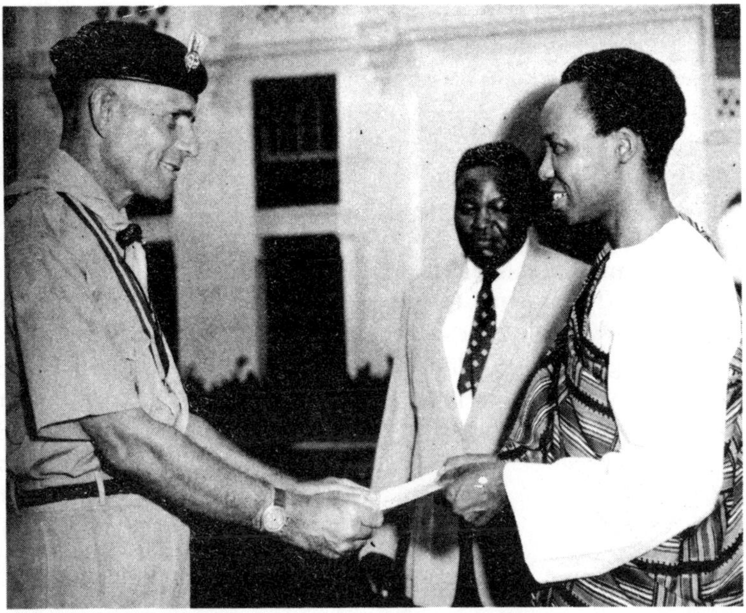

Above, Chief Scout of Tanzania: the Author receives his warrant from the President of the Republic. (Photo: Tanzania Information Services.) *Below,* our inter-racial patrol at Nkana, Zambia.

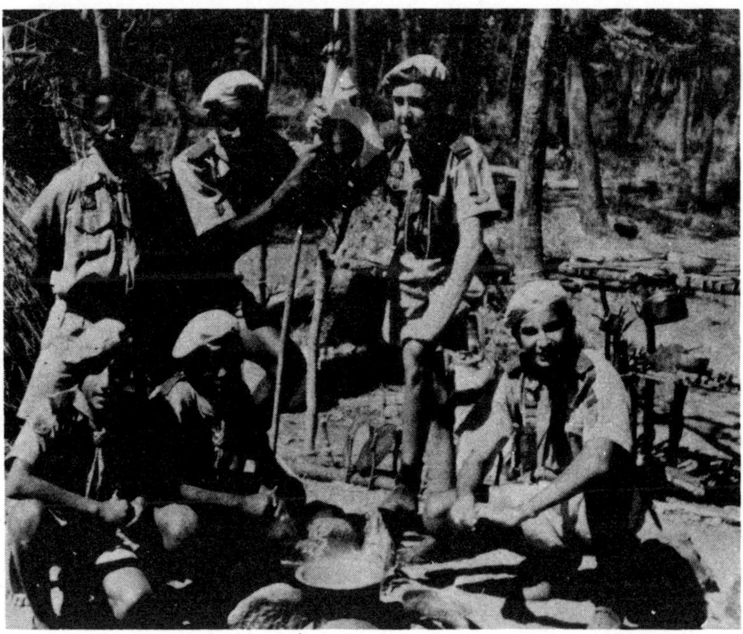

patrols carried their songs into all parts of Tanganyika, where they were taken up by the schools, then by the villages, and finally by the political movement for independence. Scouting has something to answer for.

After these two Jamborees local people began saying "The Doctor has taken the Scouts here and there—he won't be content till he's taken them to England." This duly came to pass in 1957 when the Jubilee Jamboree of Scouting was held at Sutton Coldfield and we raised a contingent of thirty Tanzanian Scouts (genuinely Tanzanian, as one patrol of six Scouts was from Zanzibar). We took Africa to England, and in a vast sea of tents we camped in grass huts—which were not only a showpiece, but were definitely more weatherproof than many of the tents when the English summer came into its own.

17
A Holiday

Those long journeys on foot in my earlier days were often wearing, but at least you could be sure that you would eventually arrive. Legs rarely break down or become completely stuck in the mud, and even if a river is unfordable, you can at least swim across it. With a car, however, there is no such certainty.

One St. Benedict's day ay Mnero, being a holiday we were having a welcome rest from routine work and hoping there would be no emergencies. At 10 a.m., however, a messenger arrived from Lukuledi, forty miles away, to say the Brother-carpenter was seriously ill, and would I go at once. The rains were then at their worst, but there was no alternative to taking the ambulance and hoping for the best. Four of the Scouts thought it would be good fun to come too, as they had no school that day. Afterwards I was thankful that they did.

The first twenty miles of the journey as far as Nachingwea, were not too bad, but two miles out of the town we ran down a hill and found at the bottom that a stream had washed away the bridge. The only way to pass was to cut through the bush and ford the stream higher up. This we did, slowly and tediously, cutting trees and bushes, pushing and pulling, and endlessly wallowing in the mud. However, when we were only about fifty yards short of rejoining the road, we became completely bogged down and could move no further. Luckily a gang of fifty men were building the groundnut railway close by, so we begged their help, and for a reasonably small consideration they all pulled on our tow rope and soon had us out. It was now about 2 p.m. and we were very hot and smothered in mud and sweat, not to mention the insects. We hurried on over a rough but passable road, and by 2.30 had reached Lukuledi. To our great surprise the patient himself came to the door to greet us. He explained cheerfully that he had only had an itching rash on his bottom, and anyway he had been given some good ointment by the dispensary.

We were glad to accept some coffee and bread, as we had missed our lunch, and then hastened on our way. To return the way we had come was out of the question: the railway gang would be leaving work at 3 p.m. and without their help we should never get through the bush again. We must go the long way round, through Ndanda. However, after only three miles we came to a flooded valley, where a young man was wading through water up to his hips. No car could possibly pass, so we turned back to Lukuledi again. There the Brothers assured us that the still longer road to Ndanda, through Masasi, was passable, so once more we set off. We splashed along quite well for about five miles, but then found another bridge washed away. It was only a small stream, and the water had gone down, so we decided to take the car through. Unfortunately, however, the stream was narrow and the banks steep, so having got the front wheels down onto the bed of the stream the front bumper fouled the opposite bank and we had to work hard digging and jacking to get it free. By the time the front was clear and the back wheels down, the tail of the ambulance had fouled the near bank, so more digging and jacking was necessary. While we were thus occupied the rain started, and the watery daylight began to fade. At last, tired and wet, and just as the last light was fading we had the car safely on the other side. We piled on board, I switched on the headlights, and drove straight into a bottomless slough! All four wheels sank axle-deep in a moment, the rain was pouring down, and it was now quite dark. We had had it.

We shut the windows against the mosquitoes, ate some supper off my emergency ration of biscuits and chocolate, and settled down in our seats to sleep if we could. All night long we had the shrill chorus of the frogs, rejoicing in the rain, and the silent flashing of a thousand fireflies. With the first streaks of dawn we set to to jack up each wheel in turn and stuff in logs, brushwood, bundles of grass, anything to fill up the holes. Meanwhile one of the Scouts, Amedeo again, who was also my youthful and very faithful factotum, had managed to light a fire on a dry anthill, and made a pot of black tea. This and the remains of the biscuits made up our breakfast. By the time we had all four wheels jacked up, the children were arriving at the village primary school a quarter of a mile down the road. (*Note:* how do you use a jack in liquid mud? Well, you carry a square piece of thick board, and you use this as a float, planting the jack in the middle. When the car is fairly well up, the board quietly slides away on the mud and the jack collapses. Then you start again). With the willing cooperation of the teacher we impressed the whole school and had seventy of them on our tow-rope. They pulled so well that the rope broke, and they all fell flat in the mud! However, they found this quite funny, and after we had repaired the rope they eventually shifted the car several yards before it sank in again. We jacked up once more and again they pulled. The bog stretched about a hundred yards in front of us, a sheet of mud and water with no way round. By mid-day, after endlessly repeating this process, we had at last reached firm ground again, thanked and rewarded our helpers, and set off once more. After a couple of miles we reached a hill where the road had been so badly washed away that there were huge rifts and gullies and the car was precariously perched astride them. We could go neither forwards nor backwards until we had filled in the gullies with rocks and earth. At least it was dry! On again, and after some more splashing and floundering, but not sticking, we at last reached Masasi in mid-afternoon. As we turned into the main road, heading for Ndanda, we were stopped by a car, the driver waving wildly at us. "You can't go on! The Liloya drift is washed away!" he shouted. He was the road engineer, so we had to believe him. However, he welcomed us into his camp and gave us a meal, the first proper meal we had had for two days, and beds for the night. Next morning he went off to see about repairing the drift. His men worked on it all morning, and by about 2 p.m. he told us we could try to cross. The river was still a surging torrent, crashing over the pile of rocks that was the reconstituted drift. Some half-dozen lorries were waiting on the banks not yet liking to risk it, but the ambulance being a light vehicle could probably make it. We ran cautiously down into the flood, and scrambled over the rocks, the water rushing all round and threatening to sweep the car into the pool below. Half way across we went well and truly aground on a large rock. We got into the river and started jacking up, and then the river began to rise, rather fast. It also started raining again. At last I had the chassis just clear of the rock, and a waiting lorry on the other bank gave us a quick tow, and we were across and unharmed. Off again, and a few miles further we came to another valley extensively flooded. The water was not too deep, and the bottom was firm sand, so we risked it. However, half way acrosss we went aground on a hidden sandbank, and all four wheels were off the ground though still in the water. Luckily at that moment a party of travellers on foot came by, and kindly gave us a pull. We came off the sandbank, out of the water, and by 6 p.m. reached Ndanda, having taken fifty-six hours to cover seventy-three miles.

Next morning we were about to set out, having still about sixty miles to go before we completed the "long way round", when one of the Brothers came in saying he had left early to take the Bishop to a confirmation, and had found the Lukuledi river running four feet deep over the decking of the bridge. He had left the Bishop swimming to his confirmation and come back.

We were now completely defeated and there was no way out. I told the Scouts to walk home (only about forty miles on foot) and myself retired to bed with a high fever. I eventually got home to Mnero a week later, when both the floods and the fever had subsided.

18

Training Scouters

As territorial Training Commissioner I became responsible for organising Scouters' training courses for the whole of Tanganyika. Thanks to a number of willing helpers this was not too difficult, and we were able to provide "preliminary" courses in all the main centres. In the next ten years more than a thousand Scouters went through this training, thus making it possible to open up more troops in more areas. Besides these "preliminary" courses, however, it soon became necessary to start advanced courses for the more experienced Scouters. These followed the plan of the traditional "Wood Badge" course, originally devised by Baden-Powell in 1919, and developed over the years with great success at Gilwell Park in England. I was careful to keep faithfully to B.P.'s plan, and to maintain our standards at international level, so that our Scouters could gain the Wood Badge on a level with their brothers in Britain and throughout the world. Owing to the ability and enthusiasm of several members of the training team this was not difficult, but an urgent need was a suitable training ground where these courses could be run on a territorial (and eventually national) basis.

We ran our first Wood Badge course in 1952, having previously depended on the help of Uganda and Britain for those few who could go so far. We borrowed a suitable piece of ground at Dodoma, which had the advantage of being central for Tanganyika, but the country was semi-desert and the temperature very high. Also we had no permanent facilities or equipment. However, the course went well, even though a foolish young Indian threw himself backwards out of a tree and suffered severe spinal concussion. He was lucky not to break his back, but he showed himself to have been an unsuitable choice for a course requiring both intelligence and ability, and he was not awarded the Wood Badge. Two years later we tried a second course at Tabora, which was a better site but very far from the south and east of Tanganyika, and the journey there from Mnero, nearly 1,000 miles, with half a dozen candidates in the car, was an adventure in itself. The petrol pipe burst 150 miles from anywhere, but I managed to borrow some solder from a small mission and, surprisingly, to buy some flex from the village shop, and achieved a successful repair. Later that night both lights and brakes failed, but by driving at a snail's pace with someone walking to find the road we reached another small mission and Amadeo spent half the night repairing the brakes. The missionaries, who were very kind, told us to be careful, as there was no water for the next seventy miles, so we took a good supply and leaving with the dawn arrived safely at Tabora after only two punctures. We were welcomed by John Crabbe, the local Scout Commissioner and Deputy Camp Chief, who, knowing the country, was not at all put out by our arriving nearly twenty-four hours late. The course began on time four hours later.

After that we (the training team) tried to find a permanent site, which would be suitable and at the same time reasonably accessible, and after casting far and wide we settled on a piece of ground called Bahati in the foothills of the Uluguru Mountains above Morogoro, accessible by both road and rail from all parts of the country. There were eleven acres of an old fruit garden, and a tumble-down house. However, there were plenty of trees, and abundant water from two tumbling mountain streams, which were big enough for swimming and ideal for a great variety of pioneering projects and obstacle activities. The hillside was steep but it had been well terraced, so there was room for the normal activities of thirty to forty Scouters. Behind the old house the mountains went straight up to about 8,000 feet, with rocky peaks, deep valleys and primeval rain forests, so there was plenty of scope for exploration and the traditional twenty-four-hour Wood Badge hike.

Bahati means luck, and it was truly a lucky find. The place had belonged to the heirs of the first Lord Kitchener, and they kindly allowed the Scouts to have it for the peppercorn rent of twenty shillings a year. We eventually acquired the unrestricted "right of occupancy". Meanwhile we gradually developed it as far as funds would allow, and it became so attractive that it was eventually selected for an international training course as being the best training ground in tropical Africa. I ran the first Wood Badge course there in 1955, and since then we have had courses almost annually, besides camps and other activities. The course is reputed to be tough, but most of the candidates remember it with pleasure. The place has a deep attraction, in fact a fascination, which grows with each time one comes back to it.

With the formation of the Republic in 1962 I found myself chosen as its Chief Scout, so handed over the Training Team to my old friend Robin Lamburn who, although older than I am, maintained the highest traditions of Scouter-training for the next twelve years. On his resignation, he left the Training Team in the hands of Isidor Ngunga, one of my most outstanding Scouters. The next most-senior member of the Training Team, Emmanuel Kibira, took my place as Chief Scout of Tanzania.

19
The Problems of Insanity and Paralysis

Until quite recent years, the problem of mental illness was largely ignored in Tanzania. The Lutheran Mission, with commendable initiative, had opened two asylums for sheltering chronic and hopeless cases, but with no resident doctor, and both were in the same small area (Usambara). There was (and is) also a "Broadmoor" type of institution for "criminal lunatics", but to gain admission there it was necessary to have been brought to court on a criminal charge. Otherwise, for the whole country there was only one general mental hospital for all types of insanity. This, a rather grim institution at Dodoma, was maintained by Government with a single doctor and a staff of tough orderlies. Being in the very centre of the country, it was equally far from everywhere, and was always overcrowded. To be admitted was very difficult, even for urgent cases, and even if admission was agreed upon, the prospect of sending or taking a violent or noisy patient several hundred miles in an overcrowded bus or third-class railway coach was formidable.

None of the ordinary hospitals, either Government or Mission, had any facilities for dealing with such cases, and were naturally reluctant to admit them. Consequently the "harmless" kind were simply left to roam the roads and villages (they still are), mocked by the children but otherwise unmolested. Some, of course, died of starvation or suicide, or were eaten by wild beasts while sleeping in the forest. Only when they became violent was any action taken. First they would be tied up with rope in the village. Then, if they could not be controlled, they would be handed to the police, whose duty was to dump them handcuffed in the nearest gaol. This was very unpopular with everyone, not least with the prison authorities who found them a great embarrassment. Their presence also upset the prisoners.

Only once, with the greatest reluctance, did I have occasion to invoke this procedure. This was at Lulindi when a poor old woman with cancer developed cerebral secondaries and became mentally deranged. At first she appeared harmless, but when she was found setting fire to the boys' boarding school (all thatched buildings) I felt she must be restrained. I gave her a gramme of sodium-hexobarbitone intramuscularly, and she was loaded into a hammock and carried peacefully twenty-four miles to Masasi. There she woke up in time to be put on the Post-lorry, with a police escort, where sitting on top of the luggage she made a gracious little speech to the District Commissioner thanking him for providing her with such excellent transport. Poor old Maria! It was heartbreaking to know she was going off to prison at Lindi, and as she was an incurable case I very much doubt if she ever secured admission to the hospital at Dodoma.

Another violent episode occurred at Ndanda Hospital, when one of my student-nurses from Mnero, having failed his final examination, became suddenly and violently maniacal. He was hastily confined in a small room, where he proceeded to break up three wooden bedsteads and to tear off all his clothes. He would let no one in, and violently assaulted the doctor when he tried to enter. The whole hospital was in uproar by the time the news reached me at Mnero. Could I please do something, they said. Knowing the extreme difficulty of the situation I rushed into Nachingwea and telephoned the Regional Medical Officer, who fortunately was a good friend of mine. I begged him at all costs to secure admission to Dodoma, and he not only readily agreed but promised to lay on a government plane forthwith to pick up the patient from Nachingwea. This was almost unbelievable! I drove over to Ndanda and filled the patient with sodium-hexobarbitone while half the hospital staff held him down. Then we put him in the ambulance and off to Nachingwea, where we found the plane waiting. Another student went with him as escort, and he slept soundly all the way to Dodoma and until he was safely into hospital.

Not being in the habit of consigning violent patients by air, it did not occur to me to tie him up before departure. I was only too anxious to get him safely off. Afterwards I realised with horror what might have happened if his sedation had worn off too soon and he had attacked the pilot!

A girl at Kibosho (Chapter XX) became acutely depressed and threw herself in the river. Luckily someone was coming down to wash some clothes, and pulled her out. So she went home and hanged herself. Again someone found her just in time and cut her down. Then she took a really large dose of insecticide, but she was rushed to hospital and had her stomach washed out, and survived. Her mother then decided she really must have some treatment, and took her to a local herbalist, who confined her in conditions of the utmost squalor and dosed her with the most revolting concoctions containing peoples' spittle and other disgusting ingredients. Naturally she got no better, and as soon as she was allowed home she stole a knife and settled down to cut her throat. She knew to cut at the side, not in front, but the knife must have been very blunt. "I cut, and I cut, and I cut!" she told me afterwards, but although she made a very large wound she failed to sever the carotid vessels. She was caught at it, and brought to hospital, where I sewed her up. I dosed her with anti-depressants, and encouraged her to tell me her story, which she did at great length. This probably did her good, but I formed the opinion that she was a tough case, and her mother too was a problem in her own right.

A well-known and popular teacher also became acutely depressed. He was badly disturbed and refused all food. He was eventually taken before the magistrate, already weak from starvation, but the magistrate, instead of referring him to the doctor, simply committed him to prison, where he died. This caused a great scandal, which came to my ears several hundred miles away. I was so shocked that, having checked the facts, I raised the matter on a parliamentary question, and although it was too late to help the poor teacher, I had at least the satisfaction of having the magistrate sacked.

This profoundly unsatisfactory situation of mental patients worried me deeply, and having entered Parliament I made it my business to hammer away demanding the proper facilities for their treatment that were so urgently needed. I returned to the attack every year at Budget time, and at least Government never attempted to deny the justice or urgency of my appeal. Plans for special psychiatric units in all the larger hospitals were at last formulated, but implementation was terribly slow. However these units are now in operation in half a dozen centres—which is a beginning. Equally important, a few doctors have been trained in psychiatry and a number of nurses have received special "post-graduate" training in mental nursing. Of the first five so trained, four were selected from my former Mnero students. Among these four were the ex-violent patient—who had been cured and then passed his finals—and his escort! The escort (Benedikt Komba, R.M.N.) is now the senior psychiatric tutor in the Tanzanian Ministry of Health.

As well as by these Government steps, the situation of mental patients has now been improved by the introduction of the modern tranquiliser drugs. With an adequate stock of Largactil in the cupboard, the average general hospital is no longer afraid to admit acutely disturbed patients, and at Kibosho we treated several such with great benefit. Even where a quick cure cannot be so simply obtained, the patient can at least be controlled and pacified while negotiations proceed for admission to a psychiatric unit. It also makes the eventual transport easier. In Africa there is far more sympathy and tolerance for the mentally sick than in England, and we found our nurses very ready to co-operate with these difficult cases. Even the other patients were understanding and helpful.

Another frequent problem at Mnero was that of paralysed children due to many causes, by far the commonest being poliomyelitis. This disease is quite common among Tanzanians, and although fatal cases are rare, it causes much disability. Seeing so many children thus disabled, I began to collect them together and make a systematic surgical attack on their deformities, with the willing help of the Benedictine Brothers who made the necessary boots and caliper splints. The initial results were very gratifying, and the children were delighted. The trouble came when the child was discharged and maintenance of boots and splints became the responsibility of parents. Co-operation was extremely variable, and often bitterly disappointing. It was a question not merely of expense, which could have been overcome, but of mental attitude.

Two particularly striking cases were Selina and Francis. Selina was about fifteen, and had been crawling on hands and knees ever since infancy. She was the daughter of one of our more senior dispensers, a clever and attractive child and desperately anxious to stand up and walk. Both legs, however, were almost totally paralysed, including even some of the pelvic and lumbar muscles, with severe contractures of ankles, knees, and hip-joints. Repeated operations were necessary, but at last her legs were straight and her boots and calipers fitted. We hoisted her on to her feet and put her between the parallel bars. She could now stand with support, but walking was another matter. She was in fact simply sitting in the rings of her calipers, unable to move anything but her toes. However, she was determined to walk, and she did. She would twist her pelvis round so as to swing one leg forward. Then a twist the other way, and the other leg swung forward, and so on, little by little. All day she went backwards and forwards between the bars. Then we gave her a small bedside locker on castors as a walking machine, and in a week she had completely worn out the castors! But she was walking. At last she could leave the locker and move slowly but quite securely on two walking sticks, smiling happily. I have never seen such determination. She went home and

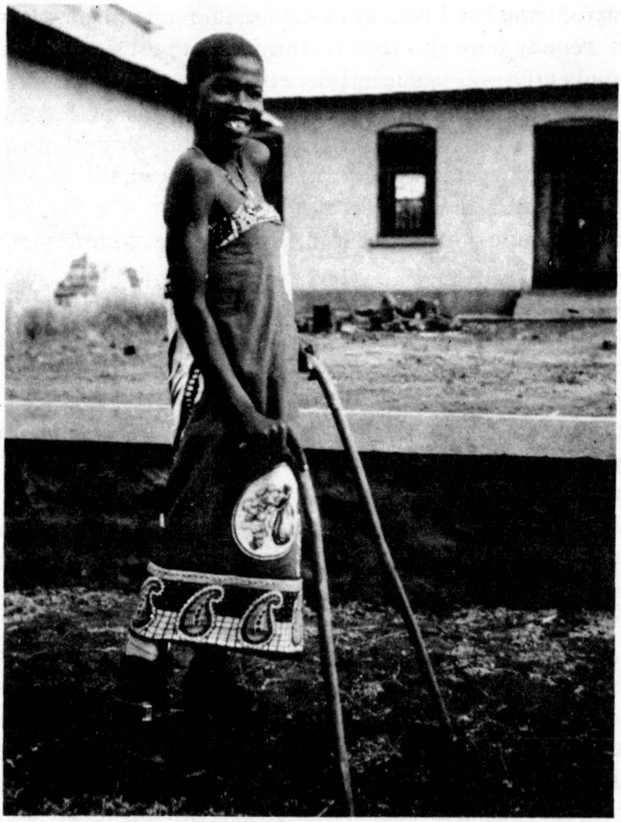

Selina vertical and triumphant.

learned a useful job, and whenever I passed her home I found her happy and active.

Francis was the opposite extreme. He also was going on hands and knees. He was not a polio case but a spastic, which is more difficult. However, he was initially co-operative, and after many weeks of operation and splinting we at last had him walking, also with the sticks. He moved around quite well, and it was a great day when he waved good-bye and tottered off on his own two feet to his home, not far away. I heard nothing of him for some time, and in those days I was busy indeed. Then, about three months later, he suddenly appeared at the hospital for some minor ailment. His sticks had gone, and he was back on his hands and knees, his legs all contracted up again. It was heart-breaking. His family background was extremely poor (his father paralytic, his mother dead, and his two aunts notoriously unreliable) so I suppose I should not have looked for the co-operation that was in fact completely lacking. There were other disappointing cases, as I have pointed out above, and eventually I became extremely cautious in the selection of children for treatment.

Another cause of paralysis seen fairly often at Mnero was spinal tuberculosis. This complication (classically known as Pott's Disease) marks a certain stage in the progress of tuberculosis in a community, and the country round Mnero had reached that stage. These children sometimes arrived severely paralysed, but with anti-tuberculous chemotherapy and a modern surgical approach, they improved rapidly. Although the operation is severe, the follow-up (simply a course of pills) being much simpler than with the polio children, the end-results were always happy. Until that time the standard treatment of such cases had always included a plaster-of-Paris "bed". However, I early had two cases which showed this to be quite unnecessary with modern treatment. In one case the patient was always demurely lying in his "bed" when the doctor came round, but only after he had been discharged cured did I discover that he had spent the rest of his time roaming round the ward! The second case was a woman whom I had treated for pulmonary tuberculosis. When she was nearly cured, a check X-ray of her chest was placed rather lower than usual, and showed two lumbar vertebrae severely diseased but quietly healing. She had had no plaster-of-Paris at all! After that I saved time, trouble and expense by consigning plaster-beds to the museum.

Peter was a happy boy of thirteen, but becoming increasingly paralysed. He was neither a polio sufferer nor a spastic: he had all the signs of a spinal tumour. I did a laminectomy in the hope of removing it, but alas, on exposing the tumour it was a diffuse one, malignant and already infiltrating the whole *cauda equina*.

Of course he remained paralysed, and one could see him gradually sinking. Every day, with a heavy heart, I would visit him and try to smile with him. He was very gallant, and there was so little I could do. At last the morning came for me to go away on leave to England. There was nothing more to be done, so I said good-bye. He held my hand with the grasp of a desperate man as I smiled with him for the last time. Afterwards my students told me how he broke down and wept inconsolably when I had gone. "Now I know I shall die", he said, "the Doctor has left me."

20

The Struggle for "Uhuru"*

Early in the 1950s the senior doctor at Ndanda, the famous Sister Thekla Stinnesbeck, suggested that I start a diocesan medical guild for our medical assistants and nurses. This was very congenial, and we soon got going. The guild was called after Blessed Martin de Porres, and was basically religious. However, it also included plenty of social, educational and charitable activities, and gave plenty of enjoyment to the hard-worked medical staff and a forum in which to air their ideas and grievances. I was a full member from the beginning, but declined to hold office. We chose as president and secretary two very senior medical assistants who filled these offices with great distinction for many years, in fact until the guild was taken over by the Episcopal Conference to establish it on a national basis as the Medical Guild of Tanzania. This operation proved too much for the patient, and the guild died, which was sad. I do not blame the bishops. If the guild had really been good it should logically have been able to extend its benefits to all parts of the country, but despite great efforts, in which the Ndanda parent branch certainly played its part, something went wrong. Its individual members, however, are still going strong in the tradition of dedicated service at which the guild aimed, and its former president, John Mpeula, R.M.A., is still working with great vigour and a superbly confident touch in charge of the outpatient department at Ndanda, the same hospital at which he began work forty years ago.

In 1958 the guild decided to have an educational outing to Dar es Salaam, which some of its members had never seen. We filled a large Landrover with those who could be spared from duty and set out on the 400-mile journey in holiday spirits. After only fifteen miles the gearbox began to break up, so we had to return at snail's pace and change it for another which happened to be lying around. We then tried again, and at last arrived safely in the great city. We saw the sights and paid various visits of educational interest. Then we saw people all streaming in one direction, and cars and lorries

---

**Uhuru* = freedom.

heading the same way decorated with green branches. It was Saba Saba* day, the seventh day of the seventh month, on which TANU, the Tanganyika African National Union, was celebrating its birth four years before. In those four years, gigantic strides had been made, and that day a fittingly large rally was being held in, or rather *outside,* the capital—outside to avoid difficulty with the police. We stuck a green branch in the Landrover and followed. We found the rally on the old aerodrome, a vast arena flanked by little hills stiff with police of every rank, field-glasses, riot-cars and all. The turnout was impressive, a huge concourse spreading out far around the little platform on which stood the modest figure of Julius Nyerere, the founder and inspired leader of the party, speaking for the nation yet to be. The crowd was quiet, completely orderly, but determined. I think the police had a dull afternoon.

Driving back to the Benedictines' town house, where we were staying, we met one of the Fathers. He looked at the green branch in shocked surprise. "You should never have put that thing up", he said, "you'll get the Mission a bad name!" I failed to see why the Mission should not support legitimate aspirations to independence, but as we had already reached home the damage, if any, was done, and I saw no harm now in removing the branch.

The hospital at Mnero grew quietly, in buildings and in numbers, and by now I was fully extended. I had been working single-handed for nearly twenty-four years, and now had to deal with eighty beds always full, several hundred outpatients daily, a weekly leprosy clinic of 400, teaching and administration of the nursing school, general supervision of the hospital, visiting a dozen dispensaries and performing up to twenty operations a week. My day began at 5 a.m. and I was hard at it until bedtime, at about 11 p.m. It is good to be young, but it was getting rather much, and at the end of the year the Bishop agreed to give me a medical colleague for the first time. (I must make it clear that I was not exceptional; a workload of those dimensions is common in tropical Africa.) In the event this new colleague proved very temperamental, and after a year he decamped at 5 a.m. with the ambulance, and was never seen again! Fortunately the ambulance was eventually recovered. However, he had done useful work, and I was able to find a less temperamental replacement, my good friend Donald Gilchrist who continued for a time to ease the load.

Later, I was able to recruit two more very good doctors from

**Saba* = seven (cf. Sabbath).

England, one of whom, Dick Dreaper, proved ideally suited to the job, and a most loyal colleague. With a staff of three doctors we were able to give steadier and more comprehensive service to our patients, and to the students. By this time the tide was running strongly for political independence, an idea I had always supported, and TANU had at last persuaded the colonial government to hold elections to the Legislative Council. The Bishop suddenly asked me if I would stand for election—he said the local TANU leaders had approached him and asked for me. With this local backing and episcopal approval, I readily agreed, and was soon in the thick of an election campaign. A Colonial official visited the Bishop and threatened what would happen to the Mission if I were allowed to take part in a series of Nationalist election meetings being organised by a strong TANU team, headed by the Chairman (now President of Tanzania), whom he described as "that bunch of crooks". The Bishop declined to be rattled. The campaign went ahead, and so overwhelming was the support for TANU that I, like many others, was returned unopposed. So began a new and fascinating activity which, taking origin from medical mission work, has continued to blend harmoniously with it and has in fact proved a logical development of it.

Work on the Legislative Council was stimulating. We, the elected members, promptly formed ourselves into a vigorous opposition, the Government benches being filled by *ex-officio* and nominated members. We kept up a relentless criticism of all Government legislation, but of course our main theme was the demand for independence without delay. When the annual budget debate came round we mounted a skilfully concerted attack, each member taking a particular sector of expenditure and between us demolishing the Government's inadequate and unrealistic proposals. The Colonial press could not withhold its admiration, and ran an encouraging leader headed "The Voice of the Opposition".

The Government was taken by surprise at the seriousness of purpose and determination of the opposition, made the more effective by comprising all three races, and although they maintained their numerical majority in the Council (by nominating as many members as necessary), they were soon obliged to yield to pressure on many points. After eighteen months of this we demanded, and were granted, new elections on a more realistic basis, with the concession of responsible government.

The number of constituencies was now greatly increased, to give every administrative district one Member, but in addition districts with a large number of European or Asian inhabitants were allowed a second Member of that particular race. I was promptly sent by TANU to contest the nearest district with a European population, namely Mbeya. It looked well enough on the map, but actually it was over 600 miles away, and so I began a mammoth exercise in commuting which was to keep me busy for the next five years. Of the road 100 miles were deep sand, which infiltrated the engine of one car and finished the bearings. Another 150 miles was over the mountains, narrow, steep and incredibly rough, where on one trip we broke two springs at once and had to share out the leaves of our only spare spring between them, and on another the universal joint disintegrated and David, my young companion, and I crawled about the road picking up the bits. We eventually reconstituted the joint using insulation tape, and in great trepidation crawled cautiously to the next town some 80 miles ahead.

Another time, I was returning from Mbeya to Dar es Salaam for a political conference, and had filled up the car with local politicians, including a well-known women's leader, the late Binti Matola. About half-way to Dar es Salaam we were cruising along at 50 m.p.h. when we saw a huge bull kudu standing on a small anthill beside the road. It was the biggest kudu I had ever seen, and a fine sight. "Oh!" said Binti Matola, "*look* at that animal!" We all looked, and at that moment "that animal" suddenly dropped off its anthill and began quietly to cross the road. This was unusual, as wild animals by the roadside, unlike hens, normally either stand still or run away from the road. There was no time to do anything, and to hit a bull kudu at 50 m.p.h. could completely wreck a car. At the very last moment the kudu suddenly appeared to see the car, and made the most amazing leap, completely clearing the bonnet of the car and crashing in the opposite ditch. Unfortunately I had a large sun-visor fitted above the wind-screen, and the kudu's hind leg caught this in passing, tore it off and fell wrapped up in it. We pulled up, and I ran back with a heavy tyre-lever to finish off the injured animal, which had smashed a leg. As I approached I saw why the kudu had not seen us sooner: he had only one eye and the blind one had been towards us. Also one horn was missing, and the other was festooned with old wire. He must have been in serious trouble at some time. Seeing me coming with the tyre-lever he now made a convulsive effort to rise, and hobbled off on three legs.

However, just then a party of travellers approached on foot, and with shouts of "Nyama!" (meat) they rushed after him with spears and machetes. I don't think he can have lasted long.

Actually getting elected at Mbeya was not so easy. There was a loyal mass of TANU supporters ready to vote for me, but before they could do so I had to be nominated, which required the signatures of thirty-five voters, of whom twenty-five had to be European. Unfortunately I was a complete stranger to the place, and my opponent, a local settler, had been round first and by various means had neutralised nearly all the available European nominators. I had several days' hard work pursuing every European voter I could find, and at last had twenty-four names. Only on the last possible day did I get the twenty-fifth from an ancient recluse in the bush who signed very readily. As soon as my opponent heard of this he rushed out with his car and brought the ancient into town, virtually by force. He met me in the street in a rage, and tried to convince me that the ancient was a simpleton and that I had unfairly influenced him. I was unmoved. The ancient was deeply offended and protested that he knew his own mind as well as the next man. My opponent finally exclaimed "I thought at least you were a gentleman!" and rushed off, angrier than ever. Then he brought a series of petitions before the Returning Officer to have me disqualified on any one of five counts of irregularity, but they were all rejected. The time for nomination passed, and I was safe.

After that I addressed some enthusiastic election meetings, and on polling day the votes poured in. My opponent became more and more dismayed and finally slipped out of the back door and vanished before the count was finished. He lost his deposit. My majority was over 6,000 and for the first time in my life I had the embarrassment of being carried shoulder high by a delirious crowd of women. (The second time was even more unexpected, when some years later I deputised for the Prime Minister at a local political festival in his own constituency.)

This was now August 1960. In October we returned to the Legislative Council with seventy-one elected members instead of twenty seven. The first Tanganyika Responsible Government had been sworn in, and the fight for independence began in earnest. In the next fourteen months we achieved, first, "Internal Self Government", and finally complete independence. The pace was fast, but under the inspiring and determined leadership of Julius Nyerere it was all achieved without a shot fired or even a bloody nose. Those were intensely exciting days with the strong feeling always that we were living through history. After our more sensational triumphs we would pour out of the Council Chamber and climb on the roofs of taxis for a triumphal procession through streets packed with cheering crowds. Childish? Not really: it was spontaneous and natural. After our lesser successes we gathered in the New Africa Hotel and discussed it all over beer and with much good humour. Those parties are far off now, but not to be forgotten.

The challenge of opposition has passed, and legislation is no longer a novelty, but the seeds of real brotherhood sown in those days of struggle have germinated and permeated our Parliament with a sense of unity and mutual tolerance and respect that endures, and above all a sense of humour that keeps its feet on the ground. There is always a store of laughter just under the surface which can erupt at any moment to puncture pomposity, dissipate anger or bring the extravagant down to earth.

When we had at last achieved Independence we were able for the first time to establish a Tanganyikan citizenship. By the new constitution no one could sit in Parliament who was not a citizen, so a number of non-Africans acquired citizenship. Another larger number did not, and resigned from Parliament in consequence. For myself, I was in no doubt about this. Having been in Tanganyika nearly thirty years, living and working with and for its people, it seemed the most natural thing to do, a ratification in fact of that life-intention of service that I had accepted on first joining the Universities' Mission. I was surprised, however, and frankly disappointed to find how few Europeans in the same circumstances as mine, especially missionaries, accepted citizenship while it was freely available. Even many of those who had spent their whole lives in the country and had every intention of being buried here nevertheless obstinately retained their old nationality. It was strange.

By the end of 1962 we had become a republic and were facing the realities of economic and not merely political independence. I was happy to belong to a young nation that was quietly trying under the leadership of its first President to pull itself up by its own bootstraps.

21

The Balloon goes up, and so to my Third and Last Hospital

During all my years with the Universities' Mission I had been bound by a contract of celibacy, but as soon as I arrived at Ndanda the Bishop had made it clear that I was perfectly free to marry if I wished. I thanked him, but at that time I had no one in view, and so matters remained for some years. Then, in 1963, I began to take increasing notice of a lovely African nurse on my staff, and at the end of the year we married. From then on, at the age of fifty-seven, life took a completely new and wonderful aspect.

The years at Mnero passed busily and happily until in 1964 the balloon suddenly went up once again. A new matron had been appointed, outwardly very charming, but incorrigibly resistant to all my plans for developing the hospital, and we presently came to an impasse. I suggested to the Mother General that if the Matron were not moved there was likely to be trouble, but the Mother General made light of it. The Matron retaliated by complaining to the Father Superior. The result was a polite letter from the Bishop proposing a written constitution for the hospital. We had been running very happily for fifteen years without one, and the draft he supplied, placing everything firmly under the control of the Matron, proved quite unacceptable, and I said so. The Bishop then said he must refer the matter to the Diocesan Council, which was duly summoned. I was commanded to appear before it and so was the Matron.

The charge against me suddenly emerged: I was "forcing the pace of Africanisation" in the hospital. This was curious, for although I should have liked nothing better than to Africanise the staff, I was quite unable to do so owing to the lack of suitably qualified Africans, and I had in fact failed to Africanise a single senior post.

The councillors, all German, brushed the Bishop aside and opened fire. The first said "No African is ever capable of any responsibility whatever." The second said "No nurse who is not a nun can ever nurse with love and devotion." The third kept repeating "You want to get rid of the Sisters, you want to get rid of the Sisters . . ." The fourth said "The.trouble, Doctor, is we can't trust you!" The fifth, an old friend of mine, looked acutely embarrassed and said nothing.

After this display of ruthlessness I had no alternative but to resign on the spot. The Bishop looked very uncomfortable, and the Matron began to cry, and said "I never wanted you to go." I left with a heavy heart. Dick Dreaper resigned in sympathy, staying only long enough to prevent the hospital collapsing. At least the Bishop gave me a "golden handshake", and the Matron was eventually removed for medical reasons.

I went to dar es Salaam and met the Bishop of Mishi, Mgr. Joseph Kilasara, C.S.Sp. He said he needed a new doctor. As he was himself an African there was obviously no danger of the bogey of Africanisation raising its head again, so I accepted. He was building two new hospitals and asked me to take charge temporarily of the more advanced one, Kibosho, and start it running. I went to Moshi and had a quick look round, and then left for a long leave to introduce my wife to England before starting the new job.

Kibosho is on the southern slope of Kilimanjaro, at a height of about 5,000 feet. All Africa lay at our feet, and the snows of Kibo, the chief peak, stood above us. There was a big population all around, but their homesteads were hidden in a dense and endless plantation (their own) of coffee and bananas.

For the third time I had the task of starting a new hospital, but this time I did not have to do the designing or the actual building. The hospital had been designed by the tireless and determined African parish priest, Father Joseph Babu, C.S.Sp., and the building was being done by an African lay-brother, Brother Rafael, assisted by several thousand parishoners. They came in gangs of a hundred and worked their stint; then another hundred took over. They terraced the mountain-side, they quarried the stone, they carried the sand from the river, and they did all the builders' labouring— for nothing. Only the masons and carpenters were paid, and these by the same parishoners who sold their coffee to raise money. One man gave £50. It was *their* hospital, and *they* were building it. Self-reliance was the big idea in Tanzania then, but when the President of the Republic passed by he was amazed. He said it was the biggest self-help project he had seen anywhere.

When we arrived, the shell of the building was complete and roofed, and the decorators and plumbers were moving in. Actually the lay-brother, a very competent technician did the plumbing himself, and the painting was done by anyone who could hold a brush, but they made a very good job of it. The enthusiasm was tremendous. "*Our* hospital!" The building was two-storeyed, in the most solid materials with a good modern finish, most attractive and very workable. There was space for 114 beds and all the necessary facilities.

My job was to bring the buildings into line with medical requirements; the design having been made without benefit of medical advice, there were a number of adjustments that had to be made, and then I had to organise the equipment and the staffing. For equipment the Bishop received a donation of £500 from Germany, and the parish priest a similar amount from America. This covered beds and basic furniture and pots and pans, but not the more sophisticated and expensive equipment needed for the operating theatre, the X-ray department and the laboratory. As I was in England just then, I raided the National Health Service, and from three hospitals obtained enough surplus equipment (several thousand pounds' worth) to make an excellent operating unit. We had two volunteer technicians from Canada (Mary McInnis and Margaret McMillan) to man the X-ray department and the laboratory, and they likewise raised all the necessary equipment for those from their old hospitals in Canada. The actual X-ray machine was given by the Bishop.

For staffing I relied on my old African friends and pupils from Mnero and Ndanda, as up till that time the local people of Kilimanjaro had not shown much interest in nursing. As I had received a shoal of letters from nurses and others wanting to follow me to Kilimanjaro, I was able to hand-pick a first-rate staff. I had no other doctor, but an excellent Medical Assistant, Beatus Milanzi, (one of my former pupils) and Senior Nurses to take charge of all wards, the theatre and outpatients, the chief male nurse being Magnus Dunyara, another of my old pupils and a most efficient organiser who could never rest while there was anything to be done. My wife took charge of the maternity department. We recruited local girls as nursing assistants, and others gradually got themselves trained and replaced our imported staff one by one. The Canadian volunteers also trained local young men in their own technicalities so that when they returned to Canada after two years, they were able to leave both the X-ray department and the laboratory very efficiently staffed.

This wholly local effort was immensely stimulating and I was intensely happy working in such surroundings. I was of course back again to single-doctor working, so once more I was on call all day and night, and it was as well I had a house almost on top of the hospital (it was up the mountain side, higher than the hospital roof, but very close, and with a telephone) as I was working till all hours. I also had the usual chain of dispensaries to cover, though more than before (eighteen altogether), but at least I could go by car to all of them, over stony mountian roads, and the 3 a.m. start on foot was a thing of the past.

It is popular nowadays to blame African countries for building too many and too sophisticated hospitals, instead of providing the more urgently needed rural dispensaries. This may be true in some places, but Tanzania, with 1,800 dispensaries already (i.e. one for every 10,000 people) and a steady programme for building 100 more every year, hardly merits this blame. I myself, while building three hospitals, opened or re-built twenty dispensaries, and took over from time to time the supervision of thirty-three more that already existed. Wherever a nurse or midwife was available, our dispensaries included a child-welfare clinic giving prophylactic innoculations, and where possible an ante-natal clinic as well. All of them provided regular outpatient treatment for leprosy and tuberculosis, common diseases often mistakenly supposed to require special hospitals.

In the early days at Kibosho the operating theatre was not yet ready, and when in emergencies we found ourselves acutely embarrassed. Late one night a woman was brought to the maternity department well advanced in labour. She had had several healthy children (the family average at Kibosho was 10-14) but this one was completely stuck, and it was ovious that only Caesarian section, without delay, could save her and the child. We simply had no facilities then , so all I could do was to put her hastily in the car and set off for Moshi, nine miles away. It was pouring with rain, and the mountain-road was slippery with thick mud, but somehow we got down.

Arrived at the Government Hospital I made straight for the labour wards, and had my patient carried in. By now she was having terrible and frequent contractions, which she bore with great courage, but I feared that the uterus would burst any minute. The scene inside the small labour room was almost beyond belief. One labouring patient occupied the labour couch in the middle of the room, two more were on trolleys and a fourth was doing her best on the floor. Everywhere was blood, debris and odd bits of soiled linen, while two tired midwives coped as well as they could. On either side was a ward full to overflowing with recently delivered or imminent cases. There was no sign of a doctor anywhere.

My patient was also received on the floor, among the buckets and the blood, and I went to look for a medical assistant. Having found one, I tried to impress upon him the urgency of the situation. He was polite, but was not going to be rushed. He was also obviously tired, and had the whole 400-bed hospital on his hands for the night. However, he came to see my patient. One look at her, and he turned quickly to me. "I think this is an *urgent case*—I must call a doctor!" I agreed fervently, and when I was satisfied that the wheels were really turning, I went home to bed. The poor woman was eventually delivered by a successful Caesarian section as the paper thin uterus was on the point of rupture, and made a good recovery. She had a fine boy, whom she named "Deo Gratias", and I was asked to be his godfather.

It was a great relief when our own operating theatre was finished and ready for use.

The medical situation at Kibosho was very different from what I had been used to. Everyone had worms, and nearly everyone complained of stomach trouble, ranging from neurosis to cancer. High blood-pressure was common (it had been rare in the south) and rheumatic fever, in the cold damp of the mountain, was not unknown. On the other hand, our old enemies bilharzia and leprosy were hardly seen at all, nor were hernia, hydrocele and elephantiasis, which for thirty years had been my surgical daily bread. The realisation of this enormous variation in regional pathology in a single country was startling. I had been shut away in southern Tanzania all those years without realising what went on a few hundred miles to the north. As it happened, just at that time Denis Burkitt was beginning his very thorough and fascinating researches into geographical pathology, and I was pleased to be able to help him in amassing material.

Another notable difference, but easily explained, was the incidence of fractures. Around Lulindi and Mnero, on the level sandy ground, falls were uncommon, and fractures from falls especially rare. Our fractures were mostly caused by falls out of trees! On Kilimanjaro, however, the paths were steep and slippery, and a shower of rain, with the addition of too much beer, would produce a crop of broken legs, arms, spines and collarbones. Later I found the same thing in the Usambara hills, only more so as the paths were even steeper. Every day there had its quota of fractures in the small district hospital.

However one feature in common with Mnero was the large number of children who were crippled by poliomyelitis, and it was a most satisfying job repairing their deformities and making them mobile. I received excellent co-operation from two Indians in Moshi, one an engineer who made every sort of steel splint and appliance, and the other a shoemaker who made the necessary boots with equal skill. But even more important was the willing and intelligent co-operation of the parents, which is of such vital importance in rehabilitation, and which had been so sadly lacking at Mnero. When the Minister for Health visited the hospital, we were able to have a parade of cheerfully ambulant children with their parents. It was a happy day.

After we had been at Kibosho a year, we had a delightful surprise in the shape of a visit from my mother, then in her eighty-eighth year. She had very willingly let me go when I first left England, but in all those years she had always firmly resisted invitations to visit me. Something about our new set-up at Kibosho stimulated her to come, and we had an unforgettable six weeks. She was fêted by us and by the staff, our friends and the schoolchildren. She survived it all, and returned to England in triumph.

22
I Drop Anchor

Life at Kibosho was busy and very happy. After five years I felt I had done the job I had been asked to do, namely to start the hospital. By now it was running well, with the staff completely Africanised apart from myself. It only remained to find a local doctor to take my place.

Meanwhile, however, a difficulty had arisen. A large new hospital had been built only seven miles away on the road to Moshi. This hospital had 300 beds, a large staff of specialists, and free treatment for all. As the Kibosho people could only keep their hospital going by charging fees, and had only one doctor for everything, they were naturally at a disadvantage. Before the new hospital was opened I suggested to the Kibosho people that they should come to terms of co-operation either with the new hospital or with Government. There was much initial obstinacy as their spirit of self-reliance was strong, but eventually they were persuaded that it was in their own best interest to cooperate, and a scheme of integration was drawn up which has been of mutual benefit to both hospitals without disturbing the management of either. Meanwhile we found our local doctor, and I was able to withdraw smoothly. For the first time I was leaving a hospital I had started without any bitterness. They gave us a tremendous party, and we piled our few belongings onto a lorry and set off for Soni in the Usambara hills. There we found a comfortable old farmhouse. The farm had gone, but we had sufficient garden and fields to supply our food, and even enough coffee for our coffee-pot. There I dropped anchor at last.

When did I realise that I belong to Africa rather than to England? I have been asked that, but it is impossible to answer. In 1942 I wrote in a letter to England that I was becoming gradually blacker and blacker "though it doesn't show outside". The process was imperceptible, and I cannot remember when I stopped looking back to England and began to look forward with Africa. I have the happiest memories of the England that was and still enjoy visiting even the England that is, but my home is here. Well, is it? Long ago at Lulindi I painted on my lintel the words: "Here have we no abiding city", and it remains true. Heaven is our home, but I cannot feel other than at home here, with so much love on every side, not only in our family but in the street, in the bush, in the village, in the hospital, in Parliament, and even in the endless committees. The waiter in a restaurant, the ticket-collector on a train, the driver of a bus, the hostess on an aeroplane, policemen, nurses, farmers, shopkeepers, postmasters and politicians—all are old friends and hand me on with love from day to day in a life that is never lonely.

After only three years at Soni, my darling wife died, and I buried her in desolation. The love and sympathy of this host of friends was overwhelming. But all my life long I have always been a lucky man and the tale of my blessings from God is uncountable. From my desolation I was rescued by one of my old Lulindi students, herself prematurely and tragically widowed from one of my old Scouts. We married, and together we have begun to "build up the waste places", and the shattered pattern of life is wonderfully restored. Also my wife has brought me six more lovely children, so how can I grow old?

I have, however, slipped quietly out of Scouting, after fifty-five years as a Scout and ten as Chief Scout of Tanzania. It is, after all, a youth movement, and they all call me the old man, so I thought it time to go. The Scouts as such have passed into the background of national life, but they have infiltrated everywhere. They are to be found holding positions of responsibility from President, Vice-Presidents and Prime Minister downwards including ministers, principal secretaries, directors, bishops, ambassadors and managers.

The smallest (and naughtiest) Scout in the great expedition to Uganda became manager of the largest sisal estate in Tanzania, and the smallest one in the expedition to Zambia is now an Ambassador. The first patrol-leader of that first troop in the south became the most senior officer in Government. Ten of my former pupils (all Scout and Guides) have become nursing officers in charge of hospitals.

So the years have gone, and the children I knew "the other day" are the men and women now running our country. The new baby whom I was called to treat soon after my arrival in Africa is now matron of our local hospital, and the little girl who long ago came running out of the night to welcome me to her village is now my wife.

Above all, the Church has gone on quietly from strength to

strength, reaching out into every corner of the country and ever growing, a great company of ordinary men and women, led by their own African bishops and priests, leaven indeed in our young nation.

We have great problems, but greater hopes. The future is with God.

23

Epilogue: Up-Anchor again

Some years ago a friend said "I suppose you'll just go on till you drop", and I supposed I should. So when I began to retire, I felt I was perhaps rather backing out. I need not have worried: events have overtaken me with a vengeance!

After fifteen years in Parliament I had become increasingly involved in committee work, and had reached a quite ludicrous situation of being supposed to sit on no less than twenty-seven committees and public bodies, some national, some regional and some at district and ward level. Fortunately many of them rarely met, and some never. The more serious of them, and the most interesting, were a number of commissions of inquiry, which when the subject of inquiry involved travelling over the whole country, were quite fascinating. Such was the inquiry into democracy in a One-Party State, which showed clearly that democracy and the two-party Westminster system are by no means synonymous or even interdependent. It also led to several interesting developments, including the institution of fifteen National Seats in Parliament, that is, Members proposed by recognised public bodies as having wide experience or ability to represent the public interest, and elected by the assembled constituency members. I was later to be elected to one of these seats, when I moved too far from my old constituency of Mbeya to continue there, and I still hold it. Things began to get serious with the appointment of a Presidential committee to investigate public spending at all levels, for which I was again chosen. Before starting we were all warned to move into Dar es Salaam and settle there until further notice. So up came the anchor, and our lovely mountain home became only a dream and a memory. The inquiry lasted nine months and involved investigating every ministry, every department, every region, and more than half the administrative districts, during which time we travelled several thousand miles. The results of the inquiry were indeed an eye-opener, and would make a book in themselves. In fact they did, but the book is not for public consumption, so it must remain closed. I was not the Chairman, but by a curious irony the committee's report has somehow been fathered on me, and it is now known in government circles as "the Doctor's Committee". This is rather embarrassing, and may well prove more so when the full impact of the committee's recommendations is felt!

We had hardly disposed of this inquiry when the Public Accounts Committee, of which I had been Chairman for ten years, was faced with the new responsibility of investigating the accounts not only of the ministries but also of all the twenty regions. This entailed extensive travelling, so off I went again, and whenever we returned we were still tied to Dar es Salaam. Then there was yet another inquiry, into the workings of our social security scheme, and again I was appointed Chairman. We produced a fairly drastic report, which we hoped would remedy a far from satisfactory situation. It did, but the ensuing necessary legislation set up a board of trustees, and I found myself its chairman. I was now fairly tied by the nose, and settled down to accept life in the capital with its heat, its humidity and its noise. At least I now had an air-conditioned office, an efficient secretary, and control of a considerable institution.

The task facing the board of trustees was formidable. Fortunately I had some very able and quite devoted colleagues, and fairly soon the financial jungle began to show some signs of order. Before we had been at it six months, however, the five-yearly general election came along and caused a temporary diversion of activity. I stood again for the same seat, and was safely re-elected to begin my eighteenth year in Parliament. Next day, however, as I was about to sit down to Sunday lunch, I received an urgent call to State House and was there briefly informed that I was to be Minister for Health. I went back to an anxious family (who had been wondering on what grounds I was to be arrested, and whether they would see me again) and a rather cold lunch. The children said: "This is like a dream, to be a minister's children!" By the next morning I was well and truly back in harness, with a reasonable prospect of proving my friend's prognostication true.

So there I was, installed in the old German building by the sea, with its crumbling battlements and trees growing out of the roof. It is some eighty years old, and has been condemned, so we cannot get it repaired and chunks of the ceiling fall on my desk as I work (but not so far on my head). We are waiting to move one day to a fine new ministry in the new capital at Dodoma. This was the old ministry I had so often visited to beg, to protest, to argue or simply to consult, and now it was unbelievably mine. It seemed like a dream come true.

To take charge of a ministry for the first time, and at the age of seventy, was a formidable prospect, but at least it was my own subject, and the problems were only too familiar. Now for the first time I had a chance to try to deal with them as I had always thought right, and I waded in. New problems crop up like weeds, day by day, but there is no lack of variety and each one is a challenge and a stimulus to greater effort.

My permanent staff received me kindly, and in fact quite enthusiastically, and I find them keen and loyal. Outside the ministry another new experience was the Cabinet, an extension of the brotherhood I had known for so long in Parliament, enhanced by the simultaneous elevation to Cabinet rank of a number of my old friends, and vivified by the presence and leadership of our President.

In my office, even when the ceiling does not fall, there is never a dull minute. There is a daily stream of callers, from Ambassadors paying courtesy calls or coming to offer Technical Assistance (the modern euphemism for aid for the needy), through disgruntled doctors and other employees of the Ministry, to the man who comes in and says "My daughter is sick, so I have brought her to you. You are the minister of Health aren't you?" But many old friends drop in too. "Doctor, I'm so happy to see you in this chair. I had to come in and give you my congratulations". However I can't spend all my time in the office. I am responsible either directly or indirectly for 133 hospitals, 152 health centres, and 1,847 dispensaries, also sixty-five training schools for the various cadres of medical workers and nurses. So I must sometimes go out and see what they are all doing. I have always enjoyed travelling, but now it has a new aspect, either a chauffeur-driven car with flag flying, or a private compartment on a train, or first-class by air with V.I P. treatment at the airports, and all the bookings made and fares paid. It is a novel feeling after so many years of getting myself around, but I am becoming used to it, and for an old man it is not unacceptable.

Then of course there are meetings, and speeches. When I revisited my old haunts of Mnero, Masasi and Ndanda, I had to make eleven speeches in three days. People like a minister to open things—or close them—or just talk to the hospital staff. And I like to talk to them for they are the people who are really doing the work, often in the face of appalling difficulties or just plain weariness, and it is rare for there not to be one or two of my old friends among them. I meet my old pupils everywhere, and get a wonderful welcome.

Parliament, too, now has a novel aspect, sitting on the front bench (shoes, socks, trousers all conspicuous!) and forbidden to ask those penetrating supplementary questions with which I used to assail unwary ministers, or in fact to speak at all except in unswerving support of a Government motion or to defend my ministry. Question time is now slightly anxious, but questions are always answered by one's Parliamentary Secretary, and mine is both experienced and resourceful, so only very rarely do I have to get up. After six months as minister the annual budget session came along, and several weeks of anxious preparation by nearly the whole ministry culminated in my first policy-speech to introduce my ministry's estimates for the coming year.

The speech was a massive document, packed with solid facts; the loving work of many able hands; I had myself written the political parts, especially on the very hot issue of the abolition of private practice. Reading as fast as was compatible with clarity and dignity, I was through it in just two hours and with the help of several bottles of water. It was surprising and gratifying to find I had a full and attentive house throughout (everyone is interested in health and disease, and especially in medicine) and it was very well received. Fortunately the debate was short—the Speaker was anxious to pass on to the next business, and anyhow I seemed to have anticipated most of the points they had prepared to raise, so I was able (again with the able assistance of my Parliamentary Secretary) to dispose of them easily and wind up with reasonable brevity. The Committee of Supply then passed my estimates without a single query. This was much more than I deserved, as in the old days as a back-bencher one of my favourite pastimes was raising hot debates in the Committee of Supply on doubtful points in the estimates, and I expected someone to do the same to me. I had all my defences prepared, but they were never needed.

When I became a minister, many people supposed I should move into one of the ex-colonial houses in Dar es Salaam's suburbia-*in-excelsis* known as Oyster Bay. However, I saw no point in doing this, as we had built a nice little house in a village the other side of town, and there we live. As political leaders are expected to live in villages with the rest of the people this seemed the obvious place to stay. There are schools for the children and some small shops, and a good road into town. We grow our own food, and keep ducks to augment our meat supply; we are also proposing to buy a couple of cows for milk. As my wife is Chairman of the village Party branch, we cannot escape politics even at home.

Perhaps I should say something of my political activities in the Ministry, but again perhaps not, as these are essentially matters of state. Suffice it to say that most of my preoccupations add up to, or contribute to, my plan for a comprehensive national health service. We already have such a service, or at least the framework for one, but I want to develop it, streamline it, and give it a new direction. Since we are a poor country my aim must be not to spend any more money than I can help, but to make the maximum use of whatever facilities are already to hand. This includes particularly the church hospitals, which account for nearly half the medical work in the country, and in which I worked for so many years.

These hospitals are now recognised as making an essential contribution to our health service, and Government policy for some years has been directed towards their complete integration with the government service. When I first came to Tanzania these church hospitals were dependent entirely on overseas support. There was no government aid, and local contributions, though morally magnificent, were very small indeed in terms of actual cash. As the years passed, expenses mounted and at the same time overseas aid contracted. People in Europe now feel "Those Tanzanians are now independent, and claim to be self-reliant; let them do it themselves". This is fair, but in practice it is very hard. Since 1946 the Government has been increasingly subsidizing the church hospitals, which otherwise would have had to close down. Even so, most of them are still compelled to charge fees (albeit very modest ones, such as 2½p for an injection or £15 for resection of the stomach), which tends to make them unpopular. Unthinking people say "They are getting grants: why do we have to pay?" The grants, of course, cover only a proportion of the costs.

In the last few years a new step has been taken. Whenever an administrative district has no government hospital, the local church hospital is designated as the District Hospital. As soon as that is done, all expenses are met by the Ministry of Health, and in return no fees are charged. The immediate result is a great increase of work (since everything is free), but the hospitals concerned are doing their best to maintain their service and keep up standards. There are now fourteen District Hospitals so designated, and another five on the waiting list (i.e. waiting for funds). In addition two major consultant hospitals are church foundations, fully supported by Government. The contribution of the church hospitals is, however, even greater than this implies, as of our twenty-three nursing schools, all but two are based on hospitals which are church foundations. That is, the church is responsible, directly or indirectly, for the training of more than 90 per cent of Tanzania's nurses, and a more significant contribution to the country's health service would be difficult to imagine. Forty years ago, Tanganyika had not one Tanganyikan nurse.

Although I have said that I cannot give details of my plans, it must be clear that here is a field to be logically exploited, that is to mobilize fully the remaining church hospitals and dispensaries, the latter being very numerous and with very rare exceptions so far receiving no Government aid whatever. The limiting factor of any such plan is simply money.

Nowadays one hears and reads increasingly about "the delivery of primary health care to the rural areas" as if it were some brilliant new idea. It may be so in some countries, but when I remember the nurses, dressers and doctors slogging through the forest on foot even forty years ago, to run weekly "mobile" clinics (Sister Anne getting sleeping sickness and Edith Shelley leprosy in the process) or living in remote isolation to run "static" clinics, year in year out, I give a hollow laugh. Tanzanian health care may still be sparse (one doctor to 23,000 people, one dispensary to five villages, ten per cent of the population living more than 10 km. from any medical unit) but what there is has always been essentially rural, and with regard to the church health units almost totally so.

In the last ten years the amount of public money spent on the nation's health has risen from less than 6 shillings to 27 shillings per head—a notable increase but still a pathetically small sum in relation to the size of the problem. We are still dealing with more than fifty communicable diseases, six of which (malaria, bilharzia, hookworm, leprosy, tuberculosis and measles) are still public health problems of frightening immensity. Also the rise in prices makes the 27 shillings worth little more than the 6 shillings was then, and as the population has doubled since 1948, and we are committed to a continuing programme of expansion of our rural health services, the total problem grows ever greater while the resources diminish.

I may be asked "What about overseas aid?" It is true that we have received, and are still receiving, a lot from many different countries, for which we are indeed grateful, and without which we should be unable to develop our services, especially our hospitals, health centres and training schools (which have now in training a total of over 2,000 health workers—doctors and all sorts). The trouble is that every piece of development, be it a new building, a new apparatus, a new technique or a new intake of students, automatically involves an increase in running costs, and the hard fact is that almost no donors are willing to commit themselves to recurrent expenditure, except on a very temporary basis. The only notable exception is the paying or subsidising of the salaries of certain foreign experts, but as we have no shortage of manpower and are training our own experts as fast as we can, this piece of aid is self-limiting and will soon cease to count.

In many countries a minister is remote from the people, either by elevation on a pedestal, or else by a wall of security or bureaucracy. Here in Tanzania we are very democratic, and I am thankful to find that being a minister has not deprived me of normal human contacts. It is true there is always an armed policeman outside the bedroom window, and I have even had a detective planted immediately behind me in church, but I move freely and people still take me as they find me. They even stop me in the street. "I say Doctor, we are in trouble with the dispensary in our village", or "Doctor, can you help me get my daughter into a nursing school?" And in the middle of the night "Hullo doctor, my daughter is having a baby. Could you run her into hospital?" Sometimes they leave it too late, and then my wife has to deliver the baby. Being a minister's wife is not normally supposed to include village midwifery, but "Out of Africa always something new".

I find I am often still "the Doctor" rather than "the Minister", but as it is what I am used to, I like it that way.

So life goes on, more public than private, every day a full day and always "things both old and new". I have headed this last chapter "Epilogue", and I must leave it there, the anchor right up and the old ship still heading into the wind.